Contents

101 Recipes for Audit in Psychiatry

101 Recipes for Audit in Psychiatry

Edited by
Clare Oakley, Floriana Coccia,
Neil Masson, Iain McKinnon
and Meinou Simmons

RCPsych Publications

CAMBRIDGE
UNIVERSITY PRESS

University Printing House, Cambridge CB2 8BS, United Kingdom

One Liberty Plaza, 20th Floor, New York, NY 10006, USA

477 Williamstown Road, Port Melbourne, VIC 3207, Australia

314-321, 3rd Floor, Plot 3, Splendor Forum, Jasola District Centre, New Delhi - 110025, India

79 Anson Road, #06-04/06, Singapore 079906

Cambridge University Press is part of the University of Cambridge.

It furthers the University's mission by disseminating knowledge in the pursuit of education, learning and research at the highest international levels of excellence.

www.cambridge.org
Information on this title: www.cambridge.org/9781908020017

RCPsych Publications is an imprint of the Royal College of Psychiatrists,
17 Belgrave Square, London SW1X 8PG
http://www.rcpsych.ac.uk

Editors

Floriana Coccia is an honorary clinical lecturer at the University of Birmingham, and a specialty registrar in general adult psychiatry at the Barberry Centre, Birmingham and Solihull Mental Health Foundation Trust.

Neil Masson is a specialty registrar in general adult psychiatry at the Riverside Resource Centre, NHS Greater Glasgow and Clyde.

Iain McKinnon is an NIHR Doctoral Research Fellow at the Institute of Neuroscience, Newcastle University, and a specialty registrar in learning disability psychiatry at the Northumberland Tyne and Wear NHS Foundation Trust.

Clare Oakley is a clinical research worker at St Andrew's Academic Centre, Institute of Psychiatry, King's College London.

Meinou Simmons is a specialty registrar in child and adolescent psychiatry at the Brookside Child and Family Consultation Clinic, Cambridge and Peterborough Foundation Trust.

Contributors

Afia Ali, East London NHS Foundation Trust
Alvina Ali, Leicestershire Partnership Mental Health Trust
Azghar Ali, Birmingham and Solihull Mental Health NHS Foundation Trust
Meera Arun, Coventry and Warwickshire Partnership NHS Trust
Yaseem Aslam, Alpha Hospital
Padma Suresh Babu, Northern Deanery
Lucy Bacon, Reaside Clinic, Birmingham and Solihull Mental Health NHS
    Foundation Trust
Anthony Bailey, Leicestershire Partnership NHS Trust
Elena Baker-Glenn, Nottinghamshire Healthcare NHS Trust
Dave Ball, Winstanley Drive Health Centre, Leicester
Thomas Barnes, Prescribing Observatory for Mental Health (POMH-UK)
Daniel M. Bennett, Royal Cornhill Hospital, Aberdeen
Rohit Bhardwaj, Leeds Partnerships NHS Foundation Trust
Sabyasachi Bhaumik, Leicestershire Partnership NHS Trust
Asit B. Biswas, Leicestershire Partnership NHS Trust
Jim Bolton, St Helier Hospital, South West London and St George's Mental
    Health NHS Trust
Rebekah Bourne, Birmingham and Solihull Mental Health NHS Foundation
    Trust
Jenny Bryden, Royal Cornhill Hospital, Aberdeen
Nasim Chaudhry, Greater Manchester West NHS Mental Health Foundation
    Trust
Lauren Coates, Norfolk and Waveney Mental Health Foundation Trust
Floriana Coccia, Worcestershire Mental Health Partnership Trust, and
    Birmingham and Solihull Mental Health NHS Foundation Trust
Louise Cooke, Coventry and Warwickshire Partnership NHS Trust
Emma Court, Ardenleigh, Birmingham and Solihull Mental Health NHS
    Foundation Trust
Delphine Coyle, Wotton Lawn, Gloucester
Jenny Dale, Birmingham and Solihull Mental Health NHS Foundation Trust
Bethan Davies, Ardenleigh, Birmingham and Solihull Mental Health NHS
    Foundation Trust

Shoumitro Deb, University of Birmingham

Sandip Deshpande, Leeds Partnerships NHS Foundation Trust

Anupam Dharmadhikari, Birmingham and Solihull Mental Health NHS Foundation Trust

Claire Dibben, Older People's Mental Health Services, Suffolk Mental Health Partnership NHS Trust

Stewart Durairaj, Greater Manchester West NHS Mental Health Foundation Trust

Hany George El-Sayeh, North Yorkshire and York PCT

Caroline Fell, AWP Mental Health Partnership Trust, and North Bristol Trust

Linda Findlay, Kirklands Hospital, Lanarkshire

Andrew Forrester, HMP Brixton

Lisa Gardiner, Oxfordshire and Buckinghamshire Mental Health NHS Foundation Trust

Ged Garry, North Yorkshire and York PCT

Ratna Ghosh, Cambridgeshire and Peterborough NHS Foundation Trust

Gautam Gulati, Oxfordshire and Buckinghamshire Mental Health NHS Foundation Trust

Deepthi Gunatilake, Coventry and Warwickshire Partnership NHS Trust

Neel Halder, Greater Manchester West Mental Health NHS Foundation Trust

Michele Hampson, Nottinghamshire Healthcare NHS Trust

Angela Hassiotis, Department of Mental Health Sciences, University College London Medical School

Agnes Hauck, Leicestershire Partnership NHS Trust

Tracy Hobbs, Winstanley Drive Health Centre, Leicester

Borislav Iankov, St Helier Hospital, South West London and St George's Mental Health NHS Trust

Matthew Impey, Sheffield Health and Social Care Trust

Sofia Jaffer, Reaside Clinic, Birmingham and Solihull Mental Health NHS Foundation Trust

Sameer Jauhar, West of Scotland Higher Training Rotation

Josie Jenkinson, Kent, Surrey and Sussex Deanery

Hitesh Joshi, Leeds Partnerships NHS Foundation Trust

Babar Kamran, Abertawe Bro Morgannwg University NHS Trust

Nicolette Kaneza, St Helier Hospital, South West London and St George's Mental Health NHS Trust

Isu Katuwawela, Birmingham and Solihull Mental Health NHS Foundation Trust

Marlene M. Kelbrick, St Andrew's Healthcare, Northampton

John Kent, Newton Lodge, South West Yorkshire Partnership Foundation NHS Trust

Sobia Khan, Birmingham and Solihull Mental Health NHS Foundation Trust

Golam Khandaker, Avon and Wiltshire Mental Health Partnership NHS Trust

Christos Kouimtsidis, Hertfordshire Partnership NHS Foundation Trust

Shankar Kuchibatla, Southwest Yorkshire Partnership Foundation NHS Trust

Ashley Liew, Birmingham and Solihull Mental Health NHS Trust

Alice Lomax, South West London and St Georges Mental Health NHS Trust

Mark Lovell, Oakrise Learning Disability Inpatient Unit, York, and Yorkshire Deanery

Victoria Lukats, Sussex Partnership NHS Foundation Trust

Jason Luty, South Essex Partnership NHS Trust

Greg Lydall, UCL Rotation, London

Rob Macpherson, Wotton Lawn, Gloucester

Rakesh Magon, Hertfordshire Partnership NHS Foundation Trust

Cameron Martin, Tees, Esk and Wear Valleys NHS Foundation Trust

Neil Masson, West of Scotland Higher Training Rotation

Frank McGuigan, NHS Greater Glasgow and Clyde

Iain McKinnon, Northern Deanery

Mercedes Acevedo Merino, Royal Aberdeen Children's Hospital

David Middleton, Cambridgeshire and Peterborough NHS Foundation Trust

Gabrielle Milner, Birmingham and Solihull Mental Health NHS Foundation Trust

Sheena Mitchell, Reaside Clinic, Birmingham and Solihull Mental Health NHS Foundation Trust

Zeid Mohammed, Tees, Esk and Wear Valleys NHS Foundation Trust

Katherine Murphy, Leeds Partnerships NHS Foundation Trust

Barnett Musiime, Birmingham and Solihull Mental Health NHS Foundation Trust

Ayesha Muthu-Veloe, St Andrew's Healthcare, Northampton

Muthusamy Natarajan, Birmingham and Solihull Mental Health NHS Foundation Trust

Richard Nixon, Leeds Partnerships NHS Foundation Trust

Clare Oakley, Reaside Clinic, Birmingham and Solihull Mental Health NHS Foundation Trust

Isaac Ohonba, Abertawe Bro Morgannwg University NHS Trust

Amelia Orchard, Birmingham and Solihull Mental Health NHS Foundation Trust

Carol Paton, Prescribing Observatory for Mental Health (POMH-UK)

Lorraine Pauley, Cheshire and Wirral Partnership/Merseycare NHS Trust

Chris Pell, Carseview Centre, NHS Tayside

Vanessa Pinfold, Rethink

Debasish Das Purkayastha, Reaside Clinic, Birmingham and Solihull Mental Health NHS Foundation Trust

Siobhan Quinn, St Helier Hospital, South West London and St George's Mental Health NHS Trust

Danica Ralevic, Older People's Mental Health Services, West Suffolk Hospital

Vishwanath Byregowda Ramakrishna, Birmingham and Solihull Mental Health NHS Foundation Trust

Laura Ramsay, Oakrise Learning Disability Inpatient Unit, York

Krishen Ranganath, Wotton Lawn, Gloucester

Vinay Sudhindra Rao, Cambridgeshire and Peterborough Foundation Trust

Frances Raphael, South West London and St Georges Mental Health NHS Trust

Felicity Richards, Worcestershire Mental Health Partnership Trust, and Birmingham and Solihull Mental Health NHS Foundation Trust

Hannah Roberts, Reaside Clinic, Birmingham and Solihull Mental Health NHS Foundation Trust

Judy Rubinsztein, Older People's Mental Health Services, West Suffolk Hospital

Larissa Ryan, Berkshire Healthcare NHS Foundation Trust

Shoba Salanki, Calderstones NHS Foundation Trust

Rani Samuel, St Helier Hospital, South West London and St George's Mental Health NHS Trust

Ruth Scally, Birmingham and Solihull Mental Health NHS Foundation Trust

Tanja-Sabine Schumm, Kirklands Hospital, Lanarkshire

Sumit Sharma, Royal Cornhill Hospital, Aberdeen

Suraj Shenoy, Newton Lodge, South West Yorkshire Partnership Foundation NHS Trust

David Shiers, Joint National Early Intervention Programme Leads, National Mental Health Development Unit

Amber Shingleton-Smith, Programme Manager, Prescribing Observatory for Mental Health (POMH-UK)

Rehan Ahmed Siddiquee, Birmingham and Solihull Mental Health NHS Foundation Trust

Meinou Simmons, Cambridgeshire and Peterborough NHS Foundation Trust

Jo Smith, Joint National Early Intervention Programme Leads, National Mental Health Development Unit

Jayanth Srinivas, South Staffordshire and Shropshire NHS Foundation Trust

Susil George Stephen, Royal Alexandra Hospital, Paisley

Anna Stout, St Helier Hospital, South West London and St George's Mental Health NHS Trust

Vinay Sudhindra Rao, Cambridgeshire and Peterborough NHS Foundation Trust

Elizabeth Tanna, Hertfordshire Partnership NHS Foundation Trust

Ziad Tayar, NHS Tayside

Abigail Taylor, Birmingham and Solihull Mental Health NHS Foundation Trust

John Taylor, NHS Ayrshire and Arran

Katherine Telford, Derbyshire Mental Health Services NHS Trust

Madhusudan Deepak Thalitaya, Tinwoods Medical Centre, South Essex Partnership University NHS Foundation Trust

Joy Tomlinson, Consultant in Public Health Medicine, NHS Lothian

Gemma Unwin, University of Birmingham

Jon Van Niekerk, Greater Manchester West Foundation Trust

Kamini Vasudev, Northern Deanery, and County Durham and Darlington Priority Services NHS Trust

Gordon Walker, Winstanley Drive Health Centre, Leicester

Ollie White, Oxfordshire and Buckinghamshire Mental Health Foundation Trust

Anuprabha Wickramasinghe, Birmingham and Solihull Mental Health NHS Foundation Trust

Sarah Wilson, Nottinghamshire Healthcare NHS Trust

Nuruz Zaman, Bedfordshire and Luton Partnership Trust

Foreword

A psychiatrist who cannot show that he or she has been involved in audit is going to be in difficulties. Short-listing panels for the appointment of trainees at CT1 or ST4 as well as those for the appointment of consultants already look for evidence of involvement in audit before ticking important boxes and the emerging criteria for revalidation of all doctors include completion of a number of audits during each 5-year revalidation cycle. We cannot avoid audit. Yet one of the biggest current contributors to wasted trainee and consultant time in psychiatry that I can think of is the conduct of audit projects that have been poorly thought through. These often mercifully stall. But even if they stutter on, those involved suffer frustration and pain before they are able only to deliver a product that nobody really wants to hear about. Conduct of a successful and satisfying audit requires expertise – in terms of both knowledge and experience – as well as energy. Expertise in the planning and conduct of audits may be hard to access in many of the settings within which we work. In such circumstances, how useful it would be to have access to a series of recipes for audit projects that have been successfully completed by experts and whose results have been useful and interesting. This is the exact purpose of the book you are now reading. The expertise and experiences of our colleagues in all branches of psychiatry who have carried out audit projects that have worked and usefully informed practice and service design are encapsulated in a comprehensive range of easy-to-follow recipes suitable for all, from the absolute beginner to the *cordon bleu auditiste*. I congratulate the editors for their vision and energy in putting this book together and thank all the contributors who supplied them with their audits. Psychiatrists will be happy and grateful to have this book to help them through the requirements of appointment panels and revalidation. But maybe, also, once helped to identify interesting and deliverable projects, psychiatrists will no longer feel they are wasting time on audit and will get some value and satisfaction out of the process.

Professor Robert Howard
Dean
Royal College of Psychiatrists

Preface

As Professor Howard outlines in his Foreword, audit is an essential activity for all psychiatrists and will need to be evidenced for revalidation and by trainees in their Annual Review of Competence Progression (ARCP). This book aims to help ease this process by offering tried and tested recipes for conducting audits in clinical services. All the audits in this book have been undertaken by the authors but not all had been repeated to complete the audit cycle at the time of publication. While we have endeavoured to include a range of audit topics from all the specialties of psychiatry, there are some areas that we have not been able to include, as we wanted to include only audits that had been done in 'real life' and were reliant on the submissions from our contributors to achieve this.

We would like to thank all those who have contributed audits to this book, to whom we are very grateful. We hope that readers of this book will benefit from their first-hand experiences.

Clare Oakley, Floriana Coccia, Neil Masson,
Iain McKinnon and Meinou Simmons

Introduction

Neil Masson and Meinou Simmons

What is audit?

A standard definition of audit is an evaluation of a system or process. The National Institute for Health and Clinical Excellence (NICE), in *Principles for Best Practice in Clinical Audit* (2002), defines the process of audit as:

> A quality improvement process that seeks to improve patient care and outcomes through systematic review of care against explicit criteria and the implementation of change. Aspects of the structure, processes, and outcomes of care are selected and systematically evaluated against explicit criteria. Where indicated, changes are implemented at an individual, team, or service level and further monitoring is used to confirm improvement in healthcare delivery.

An important part of audit is that it is a cyclical process. Changes are made as a result of findings and then the same aspects of care are re-evaluated. Audit is a dynamic, ongoing process of review against standards and implementation of changes.

It appears that Florence Nightingale conducted the first documented clinical audit when she looked into standards of nursing staff hygiene during the Crimean War in the 1850s (Ashmore & Ruthven, 2008). It was not until the healthcare reforms of the late 1980s, however, that audit became widely integrated into modern healthcare, at least within the UK National Health Service (NHS) (Department of Health, 1989). Clinical audit subsequently became one of the six pillars of 'clinical governance', whereby NHS organisations were encouraged to introduce a variety of quality-improvement strategies within a coherent framework (Department of Health, 1997). As a result of these reforms, trusts appointed clinical governance advisors to help coordinate relevant audits. In recent years, audit has become an established aspect of clinical practice across the whole of the NHS.

The audit cycle

The process of clinical audit begins with the selection of a suitable topic. After choosing a topic, the next stages of audit are as follows: selection of standards;

1

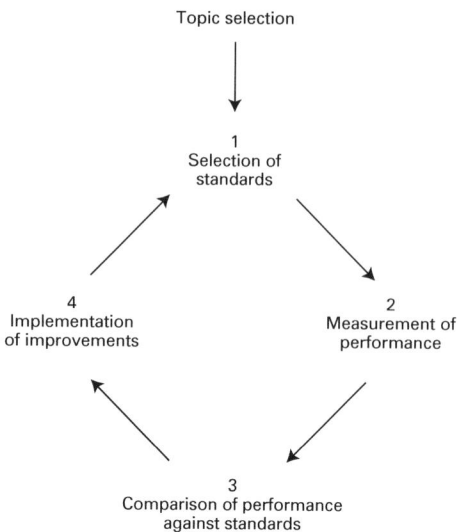

Fig. 1 The audit cycle.

measurement of performance; comparison of performance against standards; and implementation of improvements (Fig. 1). We explain the stages of the audit cycle in more detail in the next section, 'Completing an audit project' (p. 7). The stages of the audit process are repeated in a process known as the audit cycle. Re-auditing ensures that the audit continues to loop around the cycle. The steps to the successful completion of an audit project are considered in more detail in the next section.

Distinguishing audit from research

Both audit and research involve a systematic process, topic selection, sampling, data collection and statistical analysis, and both can lead to a change in practice. However, there are some general differences between the two. Distinguishing features include the following (Wade, 2005; Gould, 2008):

▶ *Purpose.* The aim of research is often to develop new practice, whereas audit examines usual practice

▶ *Relationship between the variables measured.* Research often aims to explain the relationship between variables, whereas audit aims simply to describe such variables.

▶ *Generalisability.* Research results can be applied to a wider population, whereas audit results are often specific to the service examined.

▶ *Ethics committee approval.* Ethics committees must initially approve all clinical research studies; conversely, research ethics committees often exclude audit studies from their remit.

Why is audit important?

The primary function of clinical audit is either to prove or to improve the quality of services offered to patients. Through this process, areas of good clinical practice can be demonstrated and rewarded, while areas of substandard practice can be identified, with subsequent modification of the service. Organisations often need formal evidence of substandard practice to prompt changes, and audit can be a powerful tool in demonstrating service needs. Audit can also lead to an overall improvement in the quality of health service data (Hatton & Renvoize, 1991).

Additional benefits of undertaking an audit may include improved communication between colleagues, increased professional satisfaction and the development of better administrative systems (Johnston *et al*, 2000). Psychiatrists form an integral part of services and through their contribution to audit they can directly inform best practice, and thus patient care. By contributing, psychiatrists can take ownership of their practice evaluation, and highlight service needs to managers and commissioners, which leads to them working within better systems.

Through participation in audit, psychiatrists can acquire a number of skills they will carry through their careers, as described below. In recognition of these benefits, the Royal College of Psychiatrists now requires psychiatric trainees to take part in clinical audit and the ability to conduct and complete a clinical audit is a learning outcome within the College's core curriculum for trainees (Royal College of Psychiatrists, 2009). The General Medical Council's document on revalidation is clear in stating that doctors need to continue to meet the standards appropriate for their specialty, and that audit will form an integral part of the revalidation process for doctors and will therefore be part of consultant job plans (General Medical Council, 2010). The revalidation guidance produced by the Royal College of Psychiatrists (2010) recommends psychiatrists undertake two completed audits of significant areas of clinical practice and at least one audit of record keeping in every 5-year revalidation period. With audit being a requirement for both trainees and consultants, there is an opportunity for shared working, with consultants supervising new audits and providing a longitudinal perspective on ongoing audits.

What is best practice in audit?

The Royal College of Psychiatrists' revalidation guidance (2010) includes within it the criteria and indicators of best practice in clinical audit set out by the Healthcare Improvement Partnership:

- The topic for the audit is a priority.
- The audit measures against standards.
- The organisation enables the conduct of the audit.
- The audit engages with clinical and non-clinical stakeholders.
- Patients or their representatives are involved in the audit, if appropriate.
- The audit method is described in a written protocol.
- The target sample should be appropriate to generate meaningful results.

▶ The data-collection process is robust.

▶ The data are analysed and the results reported in a way that maximises the impact of the audit.

▶ An action plan is developed to take forward any recommendations made.

▶ The audit is a cyclical process that demonstrates that improvement has been achieved and sustained.

Also, Copeland (2005) has summarised good-quality clinical audit in the following dozen golden rules:

▶ Audit should form part of a structured programme.

▶ The audit topics chosen should preferably involve high risk, high volume or high cost, or reflect national clinical audits, national service frameworks or NICE guidance.

▶ Patients and other service users should be involved in the clinical audit process.

▶ Audits should be multidisciplinary in nature.

▶ Clinical audit should include assessment of both the process and the outcome of care.

▶ Standards should be set from good-quality guidelines and backed by research.

▶ The sample size chosen should be adequate to produce credible results.

▶ Managers should be actively involved in audit and especially in the implementation of recommendations.

▶ Action plans should address any barriers to change and identify those responsible for service improvement.

▶ Re-audit should take place to establish whether improvements in care have been implemented as a result of clinical audit.

▶ Systems and specific mechanisms should be available to monitor any service improvements once the audit cycle has been completed.

▶ Each audit should have a local lead.

How can the results of audit lead to changes in practice?

The effectiveness of audit in bringing about change in practice is extremely variable, and depends on a number of downstream factors. Overall, the most successful audits are those where initial service performance was found to be poor and where there was intense feedback on that performance (Jamtvedt et al, 2006). This emphasises the importance of choosing to do an audit on a topic where change is needed and where feedback is possible. Other factors that have been found to be of importance in the success of an audit include effective training, dedicated staff, protected time, structured programmes and an environment where clinical audit is made a priority by a health board (Johnston et al, 2000; Benjamin, 2008). Several areas have audit leads or clinical audit departments which plan and coordinate audits.

Doctors are often unaware of systemic problems until they are uncovered through audit. Audits serve to highlight any deficits in how a system functions and lead to suggestions for improvements. An example at local level might be an audit reviewing sedative medication prescribed on in-patient units. If sedatives are prescribed to in-patients without regular review, many may leave hospital dependent upon that medication. Regular auditing of this practice with effective dissemination of results could help effect positive changes in practice. An example of changes in practice that occur at a national level comes from the Prescribing Observatory for Mental Health (POMH), which has conducted audit on the prescribing of high-dose and combination antipsychotics (see audit 77, p. 185), as in-patient units can compare their prescribing habits with those in wards across the UK. Wards can then work towards providing good care in this particular domain. As the POMH is now increasing the number of audits it undertakes, national comparisons will be made easier.

How can audit benefit doctors?

Audit is integrated within the everyday practice of mental health services. Many trusts employ clinical audit coordinators to oversee audits at trust level. Audits have a clear role in helping improve service provision. The process of audit also provides psychiatrists with a number of invaluable skills:

▶ *researching the evidence base for guidelines*, which can result in familiarisation with national guidelines and skills from researching relevant journal papers on the audit topic
▶ *protocol-writing skills* when putting together a protocol for implementation of the audit
▶ *planning and organisational skills* in implementing an audit within a given service framework (including assembling relevant resources, budgeting time and, often, joint working with clinical governance leads)
▶ *skills in the use of spreadsheets and other statistical tools* to process and analyse data
▶ *report-writing skills* when compiling a concise report, which may be published
▶ *presentation skills* when communicating the results of the audit to an audience
▶ *negotiation skills* with management or commissioners when seeking to implement findings, such as filling gaps within a service, or further staff training
▶ *evaluation skills* in assessing when to carry out a re-audit, and in evaluating how previous audits can be modified for different service structures
▶ *skills in developing an understanding of healthcare structures and processes*
▶ *multidisciplinary team-working skills* when the audit requires cooperation and dialogue with other staff groups.

References

Ashmore, S. & Ruthven, T. (2008) Clinical audit: a guide. *Nursing Management*, 15(1), 18–22.
Benjamin, A. (2008) Audit: how to do it in practice. *BMJ*, 336, 1241–1245.
Copeland, G. (2005) *A Practical Handbook for Clinical Audit*. NHS Clinical Governance Support Team. Available from http://www.wales.nhs.uk/sites3/Documents/501/Practical_Clinical_Audit_Handbook_v1_1.pdf (accessed October 2010).

Department of Health (1989) *Working for Patients*. HMSO.

Department of Health (1997) *The New NHS: Modern, Dependable*. HMSO.

General Medical Council (2010) *Revalidation: The Way Ahead Consultation Document*. GMC.

Gould, D. (2008) Audit and research: similarities and differences. *Nursing Standard*, **22**(37), 51–56.

Hatton, P. & Renvoize, E. B. (1991) Psychiatric audit. *Psychiatric Bulletin*, **15**, 550–551.

Jamtvedt, G., Young, J. M., Kristoffersen, D. T., *et al* (2006) Does telling people what they have been doing change what they do? A systematic review of the effects of audit and feedback. *Quality and Safety in Health Care*, **15**, 433–436.

Johnston, G., Crombie, I. K., Davies, H. T., *et al* (2000) Reviewing audit: barriers and facilitating factors for effective clinical audit. *Quality in Health Care*, **9**, 23–36.

National Institute for Health and Clinical Excellence (2002) *Principles for Best Practice in Clinical Audit*. Radcliffe Medical Press. Available from http://www.nice.org.uk/media/796/23/BestPracticeClinicalAudit.pdf (accessed October 2010).

Royal College of Psychiatrists (2009) *A Competency Based Curriculum for Specialty Training in Psychiatry*. RCPsych. Available from http://www.rcpsych.ac.uk/PDF/Core_Feb09.pdf (accessed October 2010).

Royal College of Psychiatrists (2010) *Revalidation and Guidance for Psychiatrists* (College Report 161). RCPsych.

Wade, D. T. (2005) Ethics, audit, and research: all shades of grey. *BMJ*, **330**, 468–473.

Completing an audit project

Floriana Coccia

In this section, each step in the completion of an audit is described in detail. As mentioned in the previous section, audit is conventionally described as a cycle. After completing each step of the audit process, the cycle should be repeated. This is to assess whether recommendations have been implemented and standards are now being met (or any other positive change can be recorded). As this process is ongoing, some authors describe the audit as a spiral rather than a cycle (Vasanthakumar & Brown, 1992) The re-audit is frequently omitted in clinical practice, especially where there is a high turnover of junior staff, as they are the most likely people to perform audits.

Although four general stages in the audit cycle were described in the previous section (Fig. 1, p. 2), there are more specific steps. In this section the audit cycle is broken into 11 steps. Not every step will be applicable to every audit, and some of the suggestions within this guide are just 'nice to haves':

1 Choose a topic
2 Consider forming a multidisciplinary team
3 Review the literature
4 Set standards
5 Choose an audit design
6 Collect the data
7 Analyse the data
8 Make conclusions and recommendations
9 Disseminate results
10 Implement change
11 Re-audit

Step 1. Choose a topic

Consider which area to audit

In 1966 Donabedian described three areas which can be audited in the healthcare setting: the facilities available (structure), what happens there (process) and the result for the patient (outcome). All audits are likely to fall into at least one of these categories; some may fall into two or all three categories.

The dimensions of quality of care that can be assessed in mental health audits could include access to services, relevance to need, effectiveness, equity, social acceptability and efficiency (Maxwell, 1984; Hatton & Renvoize, 1991). Trusts are now required to meet the standards of quality and safety that are set out in two pieces of legislation: the Health and Social Care Act 2008 (Regulated Activities) Regulations 2010 and the Care Quality Commission (Registration) Regulations 2009. There are 28 specific regulations, which cover the care and welfare of people who use services, infection control, the safety of premises and consent to treatment.

It is important that the auditor liaises with the local clinical governance department from the start of the audit process, as that department will be able to advise on the needs of the trust, as well as on the complexity of the audit topic to be undertaken.

Be useful

Resources in the National Health Service (NHS) are limited. Therefore the audit topic should be an important one. It is generally considered the most efficient use of resources to choose audits that evaluate issues that are high frequency, high cost, high profile and or in high-risk areas (National Institute for Health and Clinical Excellence, 2002; Copeland, 2005). An identified problem is another good area to audit, for example following an incident or complaint. Each trust will have identified a number of audits that need to be completed in any one year (these audit priorities are likely to have been identified in national policies and guidance set by the Department of Health, or dictated by the above criteria). The trust should have an audit programme that covers all the audit topics set as priorities by its clinical governance committee and this would be a useful starting place in selecting an audit topic. The trust's clinical audit coordinator will be able to advise on the audits that need to be done locally.

Be interested

Pick a topic of personal interest. Audit is perceived by many as a tedious exercise and selecting a topic of interest will help ensure that the project is completed. It will also increase motivation and make it more likely that subtle differences and variations are noticed.

Be smart

As highlighted in the introductory chapter (Fig. 1), an audit is a complete cycle. For trainees in shorter placements, completing the full cycle is not always possible. Trainees may wish to consider doing the second cycle of an audit. If the first cycle of the audit was done correctly, all the information required, the standards and data-collection documents will already be available. This would be acceptable for trainees in the early stages of training, but higher trainees, consultants and career-grade doctors should see a whole project through to completion.

Be relevant

As most doctors will now be required to develop portfolios of evidence, it would be beneficial to consider doing an audit relevant to professional needs. More junior trainees may wish to do audits on broader aspects of care that will add value to their portfolios as well as contributing to the trust's clinical governance activity.

Be counted

Registering an audit with the clinical governance department will ensure that it contributes to improved clinical care and that the work is recorded.

Be practical

The audit project will have to be feasible. There will be a limited amount of both time and resources for the task. It is better to complete a small audit than to undertake an ambitious project only to run out of time or energy before it is completed. It is also recommended that some consideration is given to the sophistication of the statistical analysis that is going to be required for the results.

Step 2. Consider forming a multidisciplinary team

The structure of modern mental health services means that most audits are likely to involve more than one professional group. If the findings are likely to affect other professionals, it is recommended that they be involved in developing the audit project from the outset. This improves the chances that any recommendations made are implemented, as all those affected feel involved from the start of the project. There is the added benefit of other perspectives on the same topic, potentially improving the quality of the audit. It also increases the pool of auditors, as other professionals may wish to assist with data collection.

The drawback to a multidisciplinary team is that resolving differences in opinion may delay the development of the audit standards and slow the process and reduce interest and enthusiasm; the audit results may be so outdated that they are of little value. To prevent such delays from occurring, it is recommended that an audit lead be appointed (Copeland, 2005) and just one or two additional members participate in the development of the audit protocol and tools.

The aim of any audit should be improved clinical care and the National Institute for Health and Clinical Excellence (NICE) therefore advises that patients and other service users are involved in the audit process (National Institute for Clinical Excellence, 2002). The most common method of patient involvement is through patient satisfaction questionnaires.

It should also be made clear from the start who is doing what aspects of the audit and what the time frame is. An audit proposal meeting, especially one involving the clinical governance department, may be helpful at this point to iron out any problems or differences of opinion early on.

The choice of project may not require the formation of a multidisciplinary team, but trainee psychiatrists should certainly discuss the suitability of the audit with their supervising consultant.

Step 3. Review the literature

Why?

A literature review should be done to identify any national recommendations that may exist, for example guidelines produced by NICE, the Scottish Intercollegiate Guidelines Network (SIGN) or the Royal College of Psychiatrists (RCPsych). There may also be published reports of audits on the chosen topic that could provide ideas for methods and standards. Where there are no published standards, research papers or reviews may assist the setting of standards for the audit project.

Where?

▶ The NICE and SIGN guidelines are available on their websites (http://www.nice.org.uk and http://www.sign.ac.uk) as well as in local NHS libraries.

▶ Health Information Resources (http://www.library.nhs.uk) (formerly the National Library for Health) allows users to search databases such as MEDLINE, EMBASE and PsychINFO, as does Scotland's Knowledge Network (http://www.knowledge.scot.nhs.uk). Both require users to register with their local library for a user name.

▶ Professional bodies such as the RCPsych (http://www.rcpsych.ac.uk), the Royal College of Nursing (http://www.rcn.org.uk) and the British Association for Psychopharmacology (http://www.bap.org.uk) have some guidelines which may be accessed online or by contacting the organisation directly. Members of the RCPsych (including pre-membership psychiatric trainees) have access to the College library.

▶ The Cochrane Library (http://www.thecochranelibrary.com) provides access to reviews and meta-analyses.

▶ National service frameworks set quality requirements for certain areas of practice and are available on the Department of Health's website (http://www.dh.gov.uk).

▶ There may be local trust guidelines on the hospital intranet site, or available from the trust's clinical governance department.

▶ If an audit recipe from this book is used, there will be standards set out and references to the relevant literature.

Step 4. Set standards

Once a topic to audit within a service has been identified, 'best practice' guidelines (preferably national evidence-based guidelines, such as those produced by NICE, or possibly local guidelines, although the latter are likely to have a smaller evidence base) can be chosen on which to base audit standards.

In audit, a 'criterion' will reflect a statement of good practice. For example, an audit criterion might be that all patients should have their weight measured. A 'standard' refers to how closely the performance of the service under study meets the given criterion. In this example, it might be '100% of patients have their weight measured'.

There are some practical problems selecting standards: it may be difficult to narrow down large sets of criteria; there may be lack of evidence in an area of practice; and the selection of arbitrary or non-evidence-based criteria will render the process less than robust (Hearnshaw *et al*, 2003). Thus, it is important to select standards carefully before the audit is begun.

Where there are guidelines available, these should form the basis of the standards. If they are not yet available, a combination of research evidence and clinical experience will provide the basis for developing an appropriate set. The standards should be written as short statements. To facilitate data collection, questions should be phrased so that adherence can be measured as either present or absent (yes/no). Where this is not suitable or feasible, a rating scale with scores of 1–5 could be an alternative. As part of the development of standards, the auditor needs to decide what qualifies as the standard being met.

For clinical data, standards are usually 100%. For other audits, for example trainees attending an induction programme, 75% might be appropriate. For a standard of less than 100% it will be necessary to decide what suitable exceptions may be applied (in the case of trainees attending induction, appropriate exceptions may be 'on night duty' or 'on annual leave').

Once the standards have been decided by all involved, the audit should be registered with the trust's audit department. In some trusts, the audit will need approval from the clinical governance committee before it can proceed. The committee will be able to highlight any potential problems early on.

Step 5. Choose an audit design

There are several factors to consider in the design of an audit.

Will it be a prospective or retrospective audit?

Data can be collected either prospectively or retrospectively and which method is chosen may depend on the resources available, the nature of the audit selected and the availability of guidelines. Table 1 outlines the differences between the two.

What information will be collected?

There is often a temptation to collect as much data as possible and 'see what we can do with it'. This is time-consuming and does not add to the quality of the audit. It also contravenes the Caldicott principles pertaining to management of patient information: do not use the information unless absolutely necessary and use the minimum amount necessary (Department of Health, 1997). Although ethical approval is not required to perform an audit, the data collection should still be performed within an ethical framework.

Table 1 Differences between retrospective and prospective audit data collection

	Retrospective	Prospective
Definition	Data collected after the event, looking back over a period of time	Data collected forward from a specified time
When appropriate	Following a major incident Where clear guidelines are available	Where no clear guidelines are available
Advantages	Most useful in the case of review of critical incidents Can provide a review of practice Can be quicker, as the information is already available	Accurate data which reflect current practice Information readily available Data not available in notes can be captured Audit staff time allocated to analysis of data
Disadvantages	Patients already in contact with service do not benefit Data required may be incomplete	Requires more data collectors Can be time-consuming

Modified from Hardman & Joughin (1998) and Copeland (2005).

The Data Protection Act requires staff not to collect or keep any information about a person or people that is not needed. It is therefore advisable to use an alternative method of identifying patients, for example a file number. This will allow the case record to be reviewed if necessary without jeopardising patient confidentiality. This advice is consistent with the General Medical Council's advice contained in its booklet *Confidentiality: Protecting and Providing Information* (General Medical Council, 2000).

Many trusts are implementing electronic note-keeping systems and these may facilitate data collection as cumbersome sets of notes do not have to be collected and all data are available online.

If the work of professionals is being audited, the aim is to assess quality in general and not to single out any individuals as performing poorly.

The rest of the information gathered should pertain to the standards set in the previous step.

How will the data be collected?

Most people use a paper-based audit tool, as this is portable and easily available. The data can then be entered into an electronic database at a later stage for easier analysis. Alternatively, the data could be directly input to an electronic spreadsheet, which would make for a speedier audit. The drawback of this method is that there is no mechanism for cross-referencing in case of errors in data entry.

How will the audit sample be selected?

The number of cases selected should be small enough to be manageable and for the data to be collected in a reasonable amount of time (if only to avoid loss of interest) but large enough to be of value. The selection can be time driven or numerical.

If it is decided to evaluate all the events that occurred within a particular time frame, 1–3 months is usually sufficient (Copeland, 2005). An example may be all patients seen in out-patient departments between January and March. This is appropriate in situations where a sample population does not remain static.

If it is decided to collect a numerical sample, the number will depend on how common the event (illness, process or treatment) is and how many parameters are being assessed. Table 2 will give an idea of the numbers required (Royal Australian College of General Practitioners, 2008). The clinical governance department will be able to assist with sample size calculations.

Table 2 Number of cases required for various categories of audit

Frequency of event	Number of clinical parameters assessed in audit		
	1–2	3–6	7 or more
Common	At least 50	20–50	5–20
Uncommon	5	5	5

In research there is great emphasis on selecting non-biased samples; this is not always possible in audit, especially where sample sizes are small. Often patient populations are selected who have similarities – similar disorders, treatments or exposure to services. Wherever possible random sampling methods should be used. Each case is assigned a number and a random-number generator can be used to select from the sample (National Institute for Health and Clinical Excellence, 2002). If another method is chosen (every second file, the first files passed on by the medical records department, etc.) this may be acceptable as long as it is clearly documented in the audit report. This will ensure that the repeat audit follows the same method.

Step 6. Collect the data

Before data collection begins, an appropriate tool should be developed. The tool should reflect the standards being measured. The simplest is a list or table presented on a single A4 sheet. There should be space for each of the following:

▶ a patient identifier – for ease of cross-referencing if needed (this should be a number rather than a name)

▶ a list of all the standards being measured (ideally with yes/no responses that can be ticked or circled).

This tool should be submitted together with the audit proposal. The clinical governance department may be able to flag up any insufficiencies and the tool will be needed for the process of re-audit.

The tool should ideally be piloted first, to pick up any deficiencies in the pro forma, for example, so that the tool can be corrected before a large amount of data has been collected. This pilot will also give an idea of how much time the data collection is likely to take. Where there are to be two or more data collectors, the reliability of data collection should be checked. Each data collector should independently extract data from the same case records and compare findings.

13

Any discrepancies should be discussed and consensus reached on how further data will be documented (National Institute for Health and Clinical Excellence, 2002).

It will be necessary to liaise with the appropriate secretary or medical records department if any patient information is needed. Sufficient time should be allowed for within the audit schedule for the records to be delivered.

Each set of data or patient record should be reviewed to ensure that it meets the inclusion criteria.

It is good practice to use one data-collection sheet per individual, clinic or ward.

Set a deadline by which time the data collection needs to be completed. If patient notes are used, try to keep them for as short a time as possible, so that clinical care is not potentially compromised. In any case, an audit is more likely to be completed if it is done in a reasonably short space of time, before any of the data collectors lose interest or move to another job.

The ethical principles mentioned above should be borne in mind in data collection.

Step 7. Analyse the data

In audit, the aim of data analysis is (generally) to compare how local practice compares with the standards set, or some sort of general level of practice in the area. Data can be analysed directly from the data-collection sheets, but most people will find it easier to enter the data into a computer-based spreadsheet.

Whereas research usually requires complex statistical analysis, audit frequently does not. If an audit does require more complex analysis, the local clinical governance department should be able to provide some support.

Most audits make use of summary descriptive statistics to answer the questions addressed:

▶ What is typical in our practice? The mean and/or median are likely to show this.

▶ How often are we meeting the standards? This is likely to be reported in the form of a rate or percentage.

▶ How widely does our practice vary? Here, the range will give an indication.

If an audit is being conducted before and after the introduction of a change, statistical tests may be required to demonstrate any true difference, one that cannot be attributed to chance alone.

Once the results of the audit have been compiled, they can be compared against the standards set earlier. It is not possible to foresee all possible outcomes at the outset of the audit. Where standards have not been met, the multidisciplinary team or auditors should discuss with each other in which circumstances it would be appropriate not to meet the standards. This will affect the denominator used; otherwise data will become difficult to interpret. There will be a range of possibilities for expressing the findings:

▶ cases meeting criteria / total number of cases
▶ cases meeting criteria / (total number of cases – appropriate exclusions)
▶ cases not meeting criteria / (total number of cases – appropriate exclusions).

Careful consideration needs to be given to how the data are presented – for example as graphs or pie charts – to demonstrate findings more clearly in the report and for the dissemination of findings.

Step 8. Make conclusions and recommendations

Conclusions are simply the summary of the results and a discussion of how local practice compares against the standards set. Before they make any recommendations, trainees should discuss the findings with their consultants.

In order for change to be implemented, the barriers to change have to be overcome. Grol (1997) recommended the following framework:

▶ The required change should be clearly defined, evidence based and presented in a way that is easy for staff to understand.
▶ The barriers to change should be identified by staff interview, team discussion and observations of work patterns.
▶ The implementation methods that are chosen should be appropriate to the circumstances, the change itself and the obstacles that need to be overcome.
▶ An integrated plan should be developed for the coordinated delivery and monitoring of the interventions. This plan should be described in the sequence in which interventions are to be made.
▶ The plan should be carried out, and progress evaluated, with modifications made to the plan or new interventions being introduced as needed.

Any recommendations should be practical and realistic. They should be presented clearly and concisely, to meet the above recommendations.

Step 9. Disseminate results

Present findings

The findings of the audit, as well as the conclusions and recommendations, should be presented to relevant parties. The presentation should include an agreed action plan that sets out any changes in practice, the staff training required and changes in standards, especially if they are local standards.

Local teaching sessions or team meetings may be appropriate venues for presenting audit findings and in many trusts there are designated audit sessions. A verbal presentation with the use of a software package like Microsoft's PowerPoint is an appropriate method for conveying the information to a large audience.

A verbal presentation is not a substitute for a written report.

Write a report

In order for an audit to be deemed completed by a clinical governance department, it will usually require a full report to be submitted. This report should detail all the steps of the audit, the standards, results, conclusions and recommendations. As outlined above, a copy of the audit tool should be included. The report should be sufficiently detailed to allow the audit to be repeated by another person in the next phase of the audit.

A copy of an audit report should always be kept in a portfolio, as it will be needed as evidence in annual reviews and appraisals.

Get published

It may be appropriate to share the findings with other services. This would be a valuable addition to any curriculum vitae. The simplest way to achieve these ends is with a poster presentation at a local, national or international conference. Each faculty within the RCPsych holds an annual conference with poster presentations. The College's annual meeting also has a display of different posters on each of its 4 days. Some of the RCPsych divisions hold audit competitions for trainees and new consultants and require the submission of an abstract and oral presentation at one of the divisional meetings.

A paper based on an audit is unlikely to be accepted for publication in a journal unless at least one audit cycle has been completed. *The Psychiatrist* (formerly called the *Psychiatric Bulletin*) has published many audits; *Clinical Governance: An International Journal* is dedicated to clinical governance matters, including audit.

Step 10. Implement change

As outlined above, an audit is unlikely to lead to real change unless the resulting recommendations are clear and practical; furthermore, they should be of benefit to patients through improving clinical care. Be wary of making recommendations simply for the sake of making recommendations.

There is also a tendency simply to add a checklist to complete, within the clinical notes for example. There may be a need to use process improvements as a surrogate for an actual outcome measure, especially where clinical change may be slow or small. Where this is not the case, the outcome should be measured directly and evaluations should not be reduced to a paper exercise.

It is likely that the trust's clinical governance facilitator will be needed to assist in implementing change, as the relevant committees will have to approve of the recommendations.

Interventions can be made at a number of levels. A basic level of intervention would be to disseminate results to service employees, which could be done by scheduling a team presentation or by circulating an electronic audit report. A greater level of intervention for more serious issues could start with the construction of a formal 'action plan'. This process may involve a formal consultation with patients, staff and management. A cost–benefit analysis could be used to analyse the relative benefits of a change in practice.

Berk *et al* (2003) found that recommendations were more likely to be implemented if: they relied on activity across a selection of service areas, rather than a single department; they involved mental health service departments (as opposed to non-mental health departments); and they did not require any change in staff attitudes.

In the unusual case of the measured performance meeting all standards, there may be no need to implement change for that particular audit. However, because of the changing nature of organisations, re-auditing of important topics is still recommended, to ensure standards are maintained, particularly in areas where best practice standards are crucial to patient care, for example in monitoring the physical health of psychiatric patients.

Step 11. Re-audit

Once changes have been implemented, a re-audit can determine whether the performance has improved. This is known as 'closing the loop' or 'completing the cycle'. The term 'audit spiral' is often used for repeat audits as it conveys a dynamic process of ongoing improvements. The process requires regular evaluation to ensure that standards are maintained. If the loop of the cycle is not followed through, the value of the audit as a practical tool is lost. The danger of 'one-off' audits is that best-practice standards are implemented temporarily and then forgotten about, a situation that has been called the 'atrophy and necrosis' phase of an audit (Hatton & Renvoize, 1991).

In order for the re-audit to be of value, there must be adequate time for any changes to be implemented. Six months may be sufficient if practice is meeting standards or only minor recommendations were made. Where a change in policy is recommended or there are multiple changes to be made, a delay of 12–18 months is likely to be appropriate.

If a good audit protocol and report have been prepared, a different individual can complete the re-audit. Trainees in most regions will be expected to complete a full audit loop by the end of their training. The establishment of a service-wide audit group can increase the number of audits in which the cycle is completed (Dogra, 2003).

Studies have shown that audits are not always carried out according to the full processes described above, thus not conforming to robust audit methods or established good practice (Greenwood *et al*, 1997; Nettleton & Ireland, 2000). One of the most common pitfalls is a failure to close the audit loop and re-audit.

References

Berk, M., Callaly, T. & Hyland, M. (2003) The evolution of clinical audit as a tool for quality improvement. *Journal of Evaluation in Clinical Practice*, 9(2), 251–257.

Copeland, G. (2005) *A Practical Handbook for Clinical Audit*. NHS Clinical Governance Support Team.

Department of Health (1997) *The Caldicott Committee Report on the Review of Patient Identifiable Information*. Department of Health.

Dogra, N. (2003) Auditing audit. *Clinical Child Psychology and Psychiatry*, 8(1), 27–35.

Donabedian, A. (1966) Evaluating the quality of medical care. *Milbank Memorial Federation of Quality*, 44, 166–208.

General Medical Council (2000) *Confidentiality: Protecting and Providing Information*. GMC.

Greenwood, J. P., Lindsay, S. J., Batin, P. D., *et al* (1997) Junior doctors and clinical audit. *Journal of the Royal College of Physicians of London*, **31**(6), 648–651.

Grol, R. (1997) Beliefs and evidence in changing clinical practice. *BMJ*, **315**, 418–421.

Hardman, E. & Joughin, C. (1998) *FOCUS on Clinical Audit in Child and Adolescent Mental Health Services*. RCPsych. Available at http://www.rcpsych.ac.uk/publications/books/rcpp/1901242234.aspx (accessed October 2010).

Hatton, P. & Renvoize, E. B. (1991) Psychiatric audit. *Psychiatric Bulletin*, **15**, 550–551.

Hearnshaw, H. M., Harker, R. M., Cheater, F. M., *et al* (2003) Are audits wasting resources by measuring the wrong things? A survey of methods used to select audit review criteria. *Quality and Safety in Health Care*, **12**, 24–28.

Maxwell, R. J. (1984) Quality assessment in health. *BMJ*, **288**, 1470–1472.

National Institute for Health and Clinical Excellence (2002) *Principles for Best Practice in Clinical Audit*. Radcliffe Medical Press.

Nettleton, J. & Ireland, A. (2000) Junior doctors' views on clinical audit – has anything changed? *International Journal of Health Care Quality Assurance*, **13**, 245–253.

Royal Australian College of General Practitioners (2008) *Clinical Audit – Application Guide*. Available at http://www.racgp.org.au/Content/NavigationMenu/educationandtraining/QACPD/20082010Triennium/20082010TrienniumProgramforGPs/GPformsandguides/docs/20082010ClinicalAuditApplicationGuide.pdf (accessed October 2010).

Vasanthakumar, V. & Brown, P. M. (1992) Audit spiral. *Quality in Health Care*, **1**(2), 142–143.

I. Disorders

Acute confusion: recognition
Antenatal and postnatal mental health
Attention-deficit hyperactivity disorder: provision of information
Bipolar depression: treatment
Bipolar disorder: management
Bipolar disorder: shared decision-making
Bipolar disorder: treatment
Chronic fatigue syndrome
Dementia: driving
Dementia: end-of-life care
Dementia: investigations
Depression: management in children and young people
Eating disorders: management
Epilepsy: management
Opiate dependence and pregnancy
Schizophrenia: family interventions
Schizophrenia: management
Schizophrenia: occupational achievements
Self-harm: assessment
Self-harm: assessment in children

1. Acute confusion: recognition

Jenny Bryden

Setting

This audit would be most relevant to liaison psychiatry within a general hospital, especially wards with a relatively high proportion of admissions for an acute confusional state (ACS) (orthopaedics, acute medical admissions, medicine of the elderly, etc.).

Background

An ACS is defined as acute onset of new or worsened cognitive deficit with disturbed consciousness, preferably with evidence of causation by either a medical condition or the action or withdrawal of a substance. The Royal College of Physicians' guidelines for the prevention, recognition and management of delirium in older people estimates that the condition affects up to 30% of older medical patients (Royal College of Physicians, 2006).

Acute confusion can have a range of serious underlying causes and is associated with a raised mortality rate. Confused patients stay in hospital significantly longer, are less able to comply with treatment and are less likely to return home.

Clinical recognition of acute confusion is poor, particularly for patients who become lethargic (the most common subtype). Identification of acutely confused patients is important, however, in order that they be appropriately investigated and any underlying causes treated. Among patients identified as being at risk of an ACS, the Royal College of Physicians (2006) estimates that the rate can be reduced by 30% by using appropriate preventative strategies.

Standards

Guidelines from the Royal College of Physicians (2006) recommend that:

▶ all patients aged over 65 be screened for confusion on admission, using the Abbreviated Mental Test (AMT) or the Mini Mental State Examination (MMSE)

▶ patients over 65 who are at increased risk of an ACS (older patients; the visually impaired; those with pre-existing confusion or physical frailty; those with polypharmacy, alcohol dependence or renal impairment; those who are on anticholinergic drugs or who are undergoing surgery) should be reassessed serially (the exact timing is not stipulated) with the AMT or MMSE.

The target is for all patients over 65 to be screened on admission and all high-risk patients to be re-screened by 1 week.

Method

Data collection

▶ A daily trip to the ward(s) audited was required. All patients admitted in the last 24 hours were identified.

▶ The medical and nursing notes of all patients over 65 were searched for a completed AMT or MMSE form. They were also examined to see whether the patient fell into a high-risk group as defined by the Royal College of Physicians.

▶ At 1 week, the medical and nursing notes of high-risk patients were re-examined for an AMT or MMSE form.

Data analysis

▶ The percentage of patients over 65 who had an AMT or MMSE noted on admission was calculated.

▶ The percentage of those patients who were classed as high risk in the guidelines and who had had a second AMT or MMSE by 1 week was calculated.

Resources required

People

This audit can be done by one person.

Time

This audit requires around half an hour per day of audit, and is best conducted over 3–4 weeks to accrue an adequate sample size.

Results

This audit was undertaken in an orthopaedics ward. No patient was tested using the AMT or MMSE at any point in their stay.

Recommendations

▶ An AMT form could be included in the nursing admission documents and/or in the standard hospital clerking sheets.

▶ In some specialties there are 'nursing pathways of care' for specific conditions, to which AMTs could be added at set points.

▶ Alternatively, many wards weigh patients weekly to screen for malnutrition, and AMTs could be added to this sheet in the nursing folder.

Royal College of Physicians (2006) *The Prevention, Diagnosis and Management of Delirium in Older People* (National Guidelines No. 6). RCP. Available at http://www.rcplondon.ac.uk/pubs/books/pdmd/DeliriumConciseGuide.pdf (accessed October 2010).

2. Antenatal and postnatal mental health

Rehan Ahmed Siddiquee, Clare Oakley and Azghar Ali

Setting

The audit is specific to the specialty of perinatal psychiatry yet is relevant to all psychiatrists, as well as midwives and primary care professionals. It relates to out-patients.

Background

The National Institute for Health and Clinical Excellence (NICE) has produced guidelines on the prediction, detection and management of mental illness among pregnant women (including but not exclusively concerning those with established mental illness) and also the criteria for referral to perinatal psychiatric services.

Standards

The following standards come from the NICE guidelines *Antenatal and Postnatal Mental Health* (National Institute for Health and Clinical Excellence, 2007):

▶ Healthcare professionals should ensure that adequate systems are in place to ensure continuity of care and effective transfer of information, to reduce the need for multiple assessments.
▶ At a woman's first contact with services in both the antenatal and the postnatal periods, healthcare professionals (including midwives, obstetricians, health visitors and general practitioners) should ask about:
  ▷ past or present severe mental illness, including schizophrenia and bipolar disorder
  ▷ psychosis in the postnatal period and severe depression
  ▷ previous treatment by a psychiatrist or specialist mental health team, including in-patient care
  ▷ a family history of perinatal mental illness.
▶ If the woman has, or is suspected of having, a severe mental illness, she should be referred to a specialist mental health service.

Method

Data collection

Data were collected from referral letters or referral forms received by the perinatal service. The referral letter and forms were examined to see if the following information was present.

▶ information regarding the reason for referral, e.g. reasons for suspecting a mental illness
▶ details of past psychiatric history
▶ current risk factors for mental illness.

Data analysis

The percentages of referrals that met each of the three standards mentioned above were calculated.

Resources required

People

It is recommended that two or three people conduct the audit, which is suitable for multidisciplinary involvement.

Time

Around 3–4 weeks should be allowed for data collection and analysis.

Results

The frequencies with which the different types of information were recorded in the referral letters and forms are given in the table below, for both an initial and a re-audit performed 1 year later.

	Reason for referral	Psychiatric history	Risk factors
Initial audit (n = 87)	79%	84%	88%
Re-audit (n = 68)	96%	72%	80%

Recommendations

After the initial audit, two recommendations were made:
- to redesign the referral form
- to provide training sessions for midwives.

These changes improved the services' compliance with the NICE guidelines and enabled the antenatal service to prioritise referrals to the perinatal mental health team. There was also a significant improvement in the proportion of referrals that were appropriate and gave sufficient information when re-audited 1 year later.

National Institute for Health and Clinical Excellence (2007) *Antenatal and Postnatal Mental Health: Clinical Management and Service Guidance* (CG45). NICE. Available at http://www.nice.org.uk/nicemedia/pdf/CG045NICEGuidelineCorrected.pdf (accessed October 2010).

3. Attention-deficit hyperactivity disorder: provision of information

Susil George Stephen

Setting

This audit is highly relevant in child and adolescent psychiatric services, where the diagnosis of attention-deficit hyperactivity disorder (ADHD) is common and forms an integral part of the clinical service.

Background

The guidelines on ADHD produced by the Scottish Intercollegiate Guidelines Network (SIGN) were first published in June 2001 and provided evidence-based guidance on the assessment and management of ADHD, including the provision of information to patients. The guideline was updated in October 2009; it included an information sheet about ADHD for parents and carers. The aim of this audit was to find out whether adequate information was provided to the parents and carers of children with ADHD at the time of diagnosis, as recommended by the SIGN guidelines.

Standards

Standards were obtained from section 6 (information for patients) of the SIGN guidelines for ADHD (SIGN, 2001):

▶ All patients should be provided with information regarding local support groups

▶ All patients should be provided with a catalogue of books, other publications and information available on the internet regarding ADHD.

Method

Data collection

▶ A random selection was made of case notes of patients with a diagnosis of ADHD seen by the service since June 2001 (when the guideline was first published).

▶ Telephone contact was made with the family/carers to enquire whether they had been provided with four specific types of information about ADHD when the diagnosis was made:
  ▷ books
  ▷ other publications
  ▷ websites
  ▷ local support groups.

▶ Findings were documented.

Data analysis

The percentage of patients for whom the following standards were met was calculated:

▶ information regarding local support groups for ADHD

▶ information regarding books on ADHD

▶ information regarding other publications on ADHD

▶ information regarding websites pertaining to ADHD.

Resources required

People

This audit can be undertaken by one person.

Time

It takes about 10 hours to collect data on 50 patients.

Results

The provision of information regarding local support groups, books and websites pertaining to ADHD was poor; the provision of other types of information (such as leaflets) was better.

Recommendations

▶ An additional page could be incorporated in the assessment pack for ADHD, with information about websites, local support groups and books pertaining to ADHD.

▶ Similarly, the pack could contain a few leaflets from the Royal College of Psychiatrists, such as 'The restless and excitable child', 'Good parenting', 'ADHD and hyperkinetic disorder' and 'Stimulant medication for ADHD and hyperkinetic disorder', to give to parents and carers.

Scottish Intercollegiate Guidelines Network (2001) *Attention Deficit and Hyperkinetic Disorders in Children and Young People* (Guideline 52). SIGN.

Scottish Intercollegiate Guidelines Network (2009) *Management of Attention Deficit and Hyperkinetic Disorders in Children and Young People* (Guideline 112). SIGN. Available at http://www.sign.ac.uk/pdf/sign112.pdf (accessed October 2010).

4. Bipolar depression: treatment

Jon Van Niekerk

Setting

This audit will be most suitable for adult and older-adult psychiatry services. Bipolar depression is usually treated within the out-patient department. This audit can be site specific or carried out across a trust.

Background

The depressive episodes in bipolar disorder are debilitating and on the whole they last longer and occur more frequently than manic episodes. The treatment of bipolar depression is controversial and there is evidence that using anti-depressants can cause switching and acceleration of cycling. The efficacy of antidepressants in bipolar depression is weak and yet they are widely used.

Standards

The following standards relating to bipolar depression were taken from the guideline on bipolar disorder produced by the National Institute for Health and Clinical Excellence (NICE) (2006):

▶ A patient who is prescribed antidepressant medication should also be prescribed an antimanic drug.
▶ A selective serotonin reuptake inhibitor (SSRI) should be used instead of a tricyclic antidepressant.
▶ Patients should not routinely continue on long-term antidepressant treatment.
▶ When initiating antidepressant treatment for patients not on antimanic medication, the risk of switching should be explained.
▶ Antidepressants should be avoided for patients with depressive symptoms who:
  ▷ have rapid-cycling bipolar disorder
  ▷ have had a recent hypomanic episode
  ▷ have recently experienced functionally impairing rapid mood fluctuations.

Method

Data collection

A retrospective case-note analysis was conducted. All patients with a diagnosis of bipolar disorder who had suffered a depressive episode were included. Those with schizoaffective disorder were excluded.

Medical/electronic notes were reviewed to see whether the following had been recorded:

▶ the severity of the depression – mild; moderate; severe; with or without psychosis
▶ any contraindications to the use of antidepressants – rapid cycling bipolar disorder, recent hypomanic episode or recent mood fluctuations

- what the baseline medications were (type and dose) and whether these had proved therapeutic/sub-therapeutic
- the treatment regimen (medication type and dose, therapy, other)
- whether the patient was on antimanic medication if an antidepressant had been started
- discussion with the patient of the risk of switching
- outcome of the treatment regimen (including adverse events such as a manic switch)
- subsequent treatment regimens (second and third).

Data analysis

Compliance with the above standards was calculated. Demographic data and site-specific data were obtained in order to allow comparisons.

Resources required

People

This was a trust-wide audit and was divided among three trainees at different sites, who were each randomly assigned 20–30 cases. The audit department drew up a list of patients with bipolar disorder within each site.

Time

The identification of suitable cases did take a few weeks. Review of 30 sets of case notes took around 20 hours.

Results

- There was poor documentation of risk of switching in the initiation of antidepressants in bipolar disorder.
- Antidepressants were by far the most popular first line of treatment – even for mild episodes of depression.
- Most patients continued on antidepressants once started.
- A significant minority became manic soon after initiating antidepressant medication.
- Documentation needed to improve, as the present level could have medico-legal implications.

Recommendations

- A memorandum should be sent to all medical staff reminding them of the importance of documentation of discussions regarding manic switch.
- An executive summary of the treatment of bipolar depression should be sent to all medical staff.

National Institute for Health and Clinical Excellence (2006) *Bipolar Disorder: The Management of Bipolar Disorder in Adults, Children and Adolescents, in Primary and Secondary Care* (Clinical Guideline 38). NICE. Available at http://guidance.nice. org.uk/CG38 (accessed October 2010).

5. Bipolar disorder: management

Madhusudan Deepak Thalitaya and Meera Arun

Setting

This audit was carried out in a learning disability service but would be equally relevant to any psychiatrists managing bipolar disorder within their community or in-patient population.

Background

According to the National Institute for Health and Clinical Excellence (2006):

▶ cases of bipolar disorder often remain unrecognised, resulting in suboptimal treatment and an increase in the total healthcare costs

▶ the annual societal cost of bipolar disorder in the UK is about £2 billion.

Standards

Standards were obtained from *Bipolar Disorder: The Management of Bipolar Disorder in Adults, Children and Adolescents, in Primary and Secondary Care* (National Institute for Health and Clinical Excellence, 2006).

▶ Risk assessment should be undertaken when bipolar disorder is first diagnosed, after a change in the patient's mental state and at discharge.

▶ In the management of acute episodes, antidepressants should be stopped and antipsychotics should be considered, taking into account side-effects and future prophylaxis. Lithium or valproate should be considered if symptoms previously responded to these medications, but they should not be prescribed routinely for women of child-bearing potential.

▶ Patients should not routinely continue on long-term antidepressant treatment. In the long term, lithium, olanzapine and valproate should be considered.

▶ For frequent relapses or severe functional impairment, an alternative monotherapy or the addition of a second prophylactic agent should be considered.

▶ A brief assessment of cognitive state should be carried out if there is evidence of memory impairment or suspected lithium toxicity.

▶ If a combination of prophylactic agents is ineffective, consideration should be given to referring the patient to a specialist, and to the prescription of lamotrigine or carbamazepine.

▶ Clinical state, side-effects, blood levels and early warning signs should be monitored.

▶ Discussions regarding reasons for the choice of agent and potential benefits and risks should be documented.

▶ Physical monitoring should be done after initial presentation and at annual check-up.

▶ Trusts should ensure that all clinicians have access to advice from designated specialists and the opportunity to refer to tertiary centres.

The target was that these standards were being met for all patients.

Method

Data collection

The target population included all community learning disability patients with bipolar disorder in the trust.

Data collection was done by a snapshot review of medical case notes. A pro forma was developed and piloted before implementation. The following data were extracted based on the standards above:

- ▶ risk assessment, clinical monitoring and physical health
- ▶ acute and long-term management and alternative interventions
- ▶ discussions with patients and carers and use of other agencies.

Data analysis

Compliance with the standards was analysed using spreadsheet software.

Resources required

People

One or two people should be sufficient for an average community area.

Time

In our audit, 12 hours was required for data collection and 2 hours for analysis.

Results

- ▶ Overall compliance achieved for acute and long-term management, clinical monitoring and use of alternative interventions was over 90%.
- ▶ Risk assessment at the time of diagnosis and documentation of discussions with patients and carers was identified as an area that could be improved upon.
- ▶ There could have been better compliance with annual monitoring of physical health.
- ▶ There were few referrals to specialist services.
- ▶ There was a wide variation in prescribing practices in the long-term management of bipolar disorder.

Recommendations

- ▶ Specialist risk assessment forms may be a useful tool to have in patients' files.
- ▶ Early warning signs and patients' preferences and compliance can be highlighted and documented at regular reviews.
- ▶ A separate physical health section in patients' folders might be useful to document healthcare needs at first contact as well as to trigger the annual physical health check-ups.
- ▶ Referral to specialist services should be facilitated.

National Institute for Health and Clinical Excellence (2006) *Bipolar Disorder: The Management of Bipolar Disorder in Adults, Children and Adolescents, in Primary and Secondary Care* (Clinical Guideline 38). NICE. Available at http://guidance.nice.org.uk/CG38 (accessed October 2010).

6. Bipolar disorder: shared decision-making

Kamini Vasudev

Setting

This audit will be relevant to any psychiatrists treating bipolar disorder in either an in-patient or an out-patient setting. It was originally conducted in an in-patient setting with patients admitted with a manic episode.

Background

The National Institute for Health and Clinical Excellence (NICE) recommends that healthcare professionals work collaboratively with patients to make a joint decision regarding treatment and care. Although the standards for this audit were taken from the guidelines for bipolar disorder, the principles could be applied to other disorders.

Standards

The NICE guideline on bipolar disorder (National Institute for Health and Clinical Excellence, 2006) includes the following recommendations:

▶ Healthcare professionals should fully involve patients in decisions about their treatment and care, and determine treatment plans in collaboration with the patient, carefully considering the experience and outcome of previous treatment(s) together with patient preference.

▶ Advance statements (directives) covering both mental and physical health-care should be developed collaboratively by people with bipolar disorder and healthcare professionals, especially by people who have severe manic or depressive episodes or who have been treated under the Mental Health Act. These should be documented in care plans, and copies given to the person with bipolar disorder, and to his or her care coordinator and general practitioner.

The Mental Health Act *Code of Practice* (Department of Health, 2008) indicates that a detained individual is not necessarily incapable of giving consent and the interview at which consent for treatment was sought, as well as the assessment of capacity, should be fully documented in the patient's notes.

Method

Data collection

The medical notes of patients suffering from bipolar disorder and admitted to hospital with a manic episode were examined for the following:

▶ documentation of discussion with patients regarding treatment options available and their preference
▶ documentation of assessment of capacity to consent to treatment
▶ reference to advanced directives if the patient was incapable of consenting
▶ advanced directives in the care plan, if the patient was currently incapable of consenting and had had previous episodes or had been detained under the Mental Health Act in the past.

For in-patient settings it might be useful to collect information on current detention under the Mental Health Act or admission to a psychiatric intensive-care unit. This might reflect on the severity of illness and may indicate whether clinical practice varies with the severity of illness, which should not be the case.

Data analysis

The percentage of bipolar patients admitted with a manic episode for whom the following standards were met were calculated:

▶ for all patients, a record of a discussion with them regarding treatment options available and their preference
▶ where this was not present, a record of an assessment of capacity to consent
▶ for patients lacking capacity who were previously known to services (i.e. who had had previous episodes or been detained under the Mental Health Act in the past):
  ▷ reference to advanced directives
  ▷ advanced directives available in the notes (with the care plan).

Resources required

People

One person is sufficient for data collection. The support of the trust's information technology department may be needed to obtain the list of patients with bipolar disorder (on the basis of ICD–10 diagnoses on discharge summaries) and secretarial support would be of value in obtaining the notes.

Time

It is estimated that 40 sets of notes will take between 12 and 15 hours to audit. It is best to limit the audit to the most recent admission.

Results

At the baseline audit, poor documentation of capacity to consent and joint decision-making was observed. The documentation had improved moderately by the time of the re-audit.

Recommendations

▶ Results and recommendations were presented at the local educational meeting and disseminated to all psychiatrists.
▶ An audit report was submitted to the trust's audit department and was made available on the trust intranet.

Department of Health (2008) *Code of Practice: Mental Health Act, 1983*. The Stationery Office. Available at http://www.dh.gov.uk/en/Publicationsandstatistics/Publications/PublicationsPolicyAndGuidance/DH_084597 (accessed October 2010).

National Institute for Health and Clinical Excellence (2006) *Bipolar Disorder: The Management of Bipolar Disorder in Adults, Children and Adolescents, in Primary and Secondary Care* (Clinical Guideline 38). NICE. Available at http://guidance.nice.org.uk/CG38 (accessed October 2010).

7. Bipolar disorder: treatment

Neil Masson, Sameer Jauhar and Joy Tomlinson

Setting

This audit is of relevance to all psychiatrists in Scotland who are involved in treating patients with bipolar disorder.

Background

The guideline on bipolar affective disorder produced by the Scottish Inter-collegiate Guidelines Network (SIGN) was last updated in July 2005 and is based on a critical appraisal of primary research evidence. The guideline separately considers treatment for mania, depression, relapse prevention, psychosocial interventions, comorbid substance misuse, reproductive health and suicide prevention.

Standards

The SIGN standards used for this audit include the following.

- In the acute treatment of mania:
  - antipsychotics, semisodium valproate or lithium should be used
  - antidepressant drug treatment should be reduced and discontinued.
- In the acute treatment of depression, an antidepressant with an antimanic drug or lamotrigine should be given.
- Intramuscular injection of antipsychotics and/or benzodiazepines should be used in emergencies for rapid tranquillisation.
- Evidence-based psychosocial interventions (e.g. cognitive–behavioural therapy, behavioural family therapy) should be available and arranged for a patient when indicated.
- Where coexisting substance misuse or alcohol problems exist, patients may be usefully managed under the care programme approach (CPA).
- In relation to suicide prevention, acute and maintenance treatment with lithium should be optimised (blood lithium level and adjustment of dose to therapeutic level).

Method

Data collection

The case notes of all patients discharged from hospital with a diagnosis of bipolar disorder over a specified period were reviewed. A standardised form was used to collect anonymised data on age, gender, diagnosis, treatment for mania, treatment for depression, medication used in rapid tranquillisation, documented need for psychosocial interventions and their availability, assessment and treatment of drug or alcohol misuse (including use of CPA) and optimisation of lithium treatment.

Data analysis

For patients with mania or depression, or those requiring rapid tranquillisation, the percentages were recorded of who were treated pharmacologically in accordance with the guideline. The proportion of patients who were referred for psychosocial interventions was also noted. Account was taken of which psychosocial interventions were available in each locality as this restricted the ability to arrange such interventions. The proportion of case notes which document the presence or otherwise of alcohol/drug misuse was noted along with the percentage of such patients on the CPA. Finally, the result of the last determination of the lithium level was noted along with the action taken if this level was not in the therapeutic range.

Resources required

People

It is recommended that at least two people conduct this audit, owing to the amount of work involved. It may be useful to collect data from multiple wards or hospital sites to increase case numbers and to allow comparisons. Administrative staff will be required to identify all patients who have been discharged during a specified period with a diagnosis of bipolar affective disorder.

Time

It is estimated that reviewing the case notes of 40 patients for this audit would take approximately 12 hours.

Results

The choice of treatment for mania, depression and rapid tranquillisation was good, as was the optimisation of lithium treatment. Carbamazepine was used for the treatment of mania in a minority of patients, which seemed clinically appropriate, although this is not stipulated in the guideline. Areas for improvement included referral for psychosocial interventions and the use of the CPA for patients with substance misuse problems.

Recommendations

- ▶ A memorandum should be distributed to all staff with details of the local protocol for rapid tranquillisation and indications for the use of the CPA.
- ▶ Hospital management should be informed of any gaps in the availability of psychosocial interventions.

Scottish Intercollegiate Guidelines Network (2005) *Bipolar Affective Disorder* (Guideline 82). SIGN. Available at http://www.sign.ac.uk/pdf/sign82.pdf (accessed October 2010).

8. Chronic fatigue syndrome

Louise Cooke

Setting

This audit may be particularly relevant in community-based and liaison services, as it is likely to be in these settings that people present with symptoms of chronic fatigue syndrome (CFS). It will also be relevant to those working in a specialist chronic fatigue service.

Background

The National Institute for Health and Clinical Excellence (NICE) (2007) states that CFS is a relatively common illness (population prevalence 0.2–0.4%), the symptoms of which can be severe and disabling, placing a substantial burden on those affected and their families and carers. To help reduce this impact there is a need for the rapid assessment, investigation, diagnosis and management of symptoms.

Standards

The investigations recommended by NICE and the ME Association in the assessment and investigation of symptoms are (National Institute for Health and Clinical Excellence, 2007; Shepherd & Chaudhuri, 2007):

▶ urinalysis
▶ full blood count, urea and electrolytes, liver function test, thyroid function test, erythrocyte sedimentation rate, C-reactive protein test
▶ glucose
▶ serum creatinine
▶ gluten sensitivity
▶ calcium
▶ creatine kinase
▶ tissue transglutaminase
▶ electrocardiogram
▶ blood pressure (patient lying and standing)
▶ score on the Epworth sleepiness scale
▶ height/weight charts in children
▶ serum ferritin level in the young.

Method

Data collection

▶ A specific (4-month) period in which to conduct the audit was identified.
▶ The medical notes of all the patients who attended a CFS specialist clinic in this period were examined to identify whether each patient had the following documented:
  ▷ confirmation of diagnosis
  ▷ confirmation of routine physical investigations, as recommended by NICE and the ME Association.

Data analysis

The percentage was calculated of all patients who attended the CFS specialist clinic for whom the following standards were met:

▶ documentation of confirmation of diagnosis of CFS

▶ documentation of physical investigations as specified by NICE and the ME Association.

Resources required

People

It is suggested that two people undertake this audit, owing to the amount of data to be collected.

Time

For a service where 16 new patients attend over a 4-month period, it is estimated that it would take 10 hours to collect the data.

Results

▶ No patients had all of the physical investigations recommended by either NICE or the ME Association.

Recommendations

▶ All investigations should be performed by the referrer before an appointment is provided for the patient to be seen in the CFS specialist clinic.

▶ A re-audit should be done and if there has been no improvement in investigations being performed then consider a 'one stop' appointment prior to the initial consultation to carry these out.

▶ Local guidelines on investigation requirements should be revised so that they are in line with national recommendations.

National Institute for Health and Clinical Excellence (2007) *Chronic Fatigue Syndrome/Myalgic Encephalomyelitis (or Encephalopathy). Diagnosis and Management of CFS/ME in Adults and Children* (CG53). NICE. Available at http://guidance. nice.org.uk/CG53 (accessed October 2010).

Shepherd, C. & Chaudhuri, A. (2007) *ME/CFS/PVFS – An Exploration of the Key Clinical Issues*. ME Association.

Acknowledgement

The original audit was by John M. O'Brien, Birmingham and Solihull Mental Health Foundation Trust.

9. Dementia: driving

Vinay Sudhindra Rao, Claire Dibben, Danica Ralevic and Judy Rubinsztein

Setting

This audit is relevant to old age psychiatrists conducting memory clinics in an out-patient setting.

Background

Guidance from the Driving and Vehicle Licensing Agency (DVLA) (2009) states that:

▶ any person who holds a valid driving licence should inform the DVLA when given the diagnosis of dementia

▶ in early dementia, when sufficient skills are retained and progression is slow, a licence may be issued subject to annual review by the DVLA.

The General Medical Council (2009) and Royal College of Psychiatrists (2005) have also published guidance on driving:

▶ It is the responsibility of doctors to advise patients when they are unfit to drive and to recommend that they inform the DVLA. This recommendation should be documented.

▶ If patients refuse to inform the DVLA, then the doctor should consider breaching confidentiality appropriately.

Standards

Based on above guidelines, the following standards can be obtained:

▶ Driving status should be recorded after the initial multidisciplinary assessment of any patient referred to a memory clinic.

▶ For patients with a diagnosis of dementia who are still driving, there should be documentation of the fact that information was given to them regarding informing the DVLA.

▶ If patients with dementia are still driving there should be documentation of a decision on whether or not to inform the DVLA.

▶ There should be documentation of action taken by the team if the patient has not acted on the advice to inform the DVLA.

▶ Expected compliance with the standards is 100%.

Method

Data collection

▶ A list was drawn up of all cases assessed in the memory clinic within a stipulated period for the audit. (DVLA procedures can be time-consuming and hence it is advisable to audit for at least 6 months in retrospect.)

▶ All documents (hand-written, computerised, printed) were examined.

▶ Exclusion criteria were set (e.g. patients who had died).

Data analysis

▶ Data were analysed using spreadsheet software.

Resources required

People

It is advisable to have at least two people involved for the data collection. This partly depends on the duration of the study.

Time

It is estimated that 100 case notes will take approximately 30 hours to audit.

Results

The first audit was done for 6 months, during which 78 people were seen in the trust's memory clinics. More than 80% had their driving status documented in their notes and 31% of those who were still driving had been advised to contact the DVLA. On re-audit a year later, 120 people had been seen, and 98% had their driving status documented, nearly two-thirds of whom had been advised to contact the DVLA. In both audits, confidentiality was breached in only one audited patient in order to disclose information to the DVLA.

Recommendations

▶ A separate heading for 'driving status' should be provided in the memory clinic assessment pro forma, to act as a prompt.

▶ Drivers with a diagnosis of dementia, or their carers, may find fact sheets helpful.

▶ Follow-up by the multidisciplinary team regarding both driving status and compliance with the advice given is extremely important.

▶ The importance of communicating with patients and carers and documenting this discussion about driving in dementia needs ongoing monitoring.

Driving and Vehicle Licensing Agency (2009) *At a Glance Guide to the Current Medical Standards of Fitness to Drive*. DVLA. Available at www.dft.gov.uk/dvla/medical/~/media/pdf/medical/at_a_glance.ashx (accessed October 2010).

General Medical Council (2009) Reporting concerns about patients to the DVLA or the DVA. In *Confidentiality: Supplementary Guidance*. GMC. Available at http://www.gmc-uk.org/static/documents/content/Confidentiality_supplementary_2009.pdf (accessed October 2010).

Royal College of Psychiatrists (2005) *Forgetful But Not Forgotten: Assessment and Aspects of Treatment of People with Dementia by a Specialist Old Age Psychiatry Service* (Council Report 119). RCPsych. Available at http://www.rcpsych.ac.uk/files/pdfversion/cr119.pdf (accessed October 2010).

10. Dementia: end-of-life care

Rehan Ahmed Siddiquee, Babar Kamran and Isaac Ohonba

Setting

This audit is particularly relevant to older-adult in-patient units where terminally ill patients suffering from dementia are placed.

Background

The Human Rights Act 1998 imposes an obligation to facilitate a good death. Despite the fact that it is difficult to define a 'good death', pathways have been developed to help patients make their final transition with the least distress. One such pathway is the Liverpool Care Pathway for the Dying Patient (Marie Curie Palliative Care Institute, 2007). It uses the National Gold Standards Framework, which is a systematic, evidence-based approach to optimising care for patients nearing the end of life. This audit is important because the Department of Health's end-of-life care strategy states that 'every organisation involved in providing end-of-life care will be expected to adopt a co-ordination process, such as the Gold Standards Framework' (Department of Health, 2008).

Standards

Standards were obtained from the Liverpool Care Pathway for the Dying Patient (Marie Curie Palliative Care Institute, 2007):

▶ recognition of the terminal stage and documentation in notes
▶ decision not to resuscitate (DNR) discussed with next of kin and documented
▶ discontinuation of non-essential drugs in terminal phase
▶ unnecessary investigations not to be carried out
▶ unnecessary monitoring of vital signs to be stopped
▶ use of medication as required to relieve distressing symptoms
▶ general practitioner informed of patient's death.

Method

Data collection

Data were retrospectively collected from medical notes, prescription cards and temperature, pulse rate and respiratory rate (TPR) charts, for all patients who had died on in-patient wards/units with terminal dementia in the past 2 years. The medical notes, prescription cards and TPR charts were examined to find documentation of the seven standards listed above.

Data analysis

The percentage of patients who had received terminal care as outlined by the guidelines was calculated and tabulated.

Resources required

People

It is suggested that this audit is undertaken by at least two people, because suitable patients may be placed on different wards.

Time

The collation of notes and collection of data from nine suitable cases in the first cycle of the present audit took one person around one working day.

Results

The end-of-life care provided to patients across the trust was of good quality. However, some shortcomings were identified in the initial audit with regard to communication with general practitioners and the continuation of non-essential medication. After circulating an integrated care pathway to all the wards and units, most of the parameters that were re-audited showed an improvement, but there were some areas of care that left room for improvement, as outlined in the table below.

	First audit	Re-audit
Recognition and documentation of terminal phase	78%	90%
Patient's DNR status discussed and documented	89%	94%
Non-essential drugs discontinued	33%	77%
Non-essential investigations stopped	0%	16%
Monitoring of vital signs stopped	22%	71%
Drugs given as required to relieve distress	66%	71%
Patient's general practitioner informed of death	0%	3%

Recommendations

▶ Training sessions should be given to all medical and nursing staff on the wards where terminal patients are likely to be nursed.

▶ An integrated care pathway should be circulated to all units where patients will be nursed.

Department of Health (2008) *End of Life Care Strategy: Promoting High Quality Care for All Adults at the End of Life*. Department of Health. Available at http://www.dh.gov.uk/en/Publicationsandstatistics/Publications/PublicationsPolicyAndGuidance/DH_086277 (accessed October 2010).

Marie Curie Palliative Care Institute (2007) *Liverpool Care Pathway for the Dying Patient*. Marie Curie Palliative Care Institute. Available at http://www.mcpcil.org.uk/liverpool-care-pathway/index.htm (accessed October 2010).

11. Dementia: investigations

Amelia Orchard

Setting

This audit is particularly relevant to psychiatrists who investigate suspected dementia, such as specialists in old age psychiatry and intellectual disability, and neuropsychiatrists.

Background

Various guidelines have been published. The National Institute for Health and Clinical Excellence (NICE) and the American Academy of Neurology recommend neuroimaging and blood tests to investigate every patient with suspected dementia. The Canadian Consensus Conference on Dementia and the Royal College of Psychiatrists recommend neuroimaging only when clinical findings point to a possibility other than Alzheimer's disease. Reasons for imaging new referrals include detecting potentially reversible causes of dementia (although the prevalence of such cases is falling) and more accurate diagnosis of dementia subtype.

Standards

The standards were obtained from the NICE guideline *Dementia: Supporting People with Dementia and Their Carers in Health and Social Care* (National Institute for Health and Clinical Excellence, 2006). The guideline recommends that a basic blood test should be performed at the time of presentation and should include:

▶ routine haematology
▶ biochemistry tests (electrolytes, calcium, glucose, renal and liver function)
▶ thyroid function tests
▶ serum B12 and folate levels.

The guideline also states that structural imaging should be used in the assessment of people with suspected dementia to exclude other cerebral pathologies and to help establish the subtype diagnosis. Magnetic resonance imaging (MRI) is the preferred modality but computerised tomography (CT) could be used.

The expectation is that all new referrals should receive a dementia blood screen and neuroimaging.

Method

Data collection

Data were collected in a retrospective review of medical notes. All new referrals to mental health services involving suspected dementia or memory problems were identified. Data collected were:

▶ age and sex
▶ whether each of the required blood tests had been performed
▶ whether the patient had a CT or MRI scan and the result of the neuroimaging (recorded in categories as Alzheimer's disease, small-vessel disease, infarct, mixed pathology, normal, awaiting scan or other).

Data analysis

The percentage of patients who had had each investigation was calculated.

Resources required

People

It is suggested that this audit is undertaken by one or two people.

Time

For approximately 50 referrals it is estimated that data collection would take around 10 hours.

Results

- ▶ Of patients newly referred with suspected dementia, 70% had received a dementia blood screen.
- ▶ Around 40% had received a CT scan.
- ▶ No MRI scans were performed.
- ▶ There were no reversible causes of dementia detected.
- ▶ The main pathologies were Alzheimer's disease and small-vessel disease (including both).

Recommendations

- ▶ All members of the multidisciplinary team who assess new patients with suspected dementia should be made aware of the need for every patient to have a full dementia blood screen and neuroimaging.
- ▶ If this is felt to be unnecessary or too difficult for some patients then this should be clearly recorded in the medical notes, with reasons stated.

National Institute for Health and Clinical Excellence (2006) *Dementia: Supporting People with Dementia and Their Carers in Health and Social Care* (CG42). NICE. Available at http://www.nice.org.uk/nicemedia/pdf/CG042NICEGuideline.pdf (accessed October 2010).

12. Depression: management in children and young people

Meinou Simmons

Setting

This audit is relevant to psychiatrists working in child and adolescent mental health services (CAMHS). It is most suited to out-patient settings.

Background

Depression has been dealt with in a variety of different ways in CAMHS. It is important to examine what happens in practice, and to monitor this regularly, according to best-practice guidelines. A 2005 guideline produced by the National Institute for Health and Clinical Excellence (NICE) attempted to standardise the approach to depression in terms of assessment and treatment according to the evidence base. More recent evidence, however, called some of those recommendations into question, including using medication as a second-line treatment for moderate to severe depression (Goodyer *et al*, 2007). However, several parts of the guideline are sound and can provide a useful benchmark for best practice in the areas of assessment and treatment.

Standards

Assessment standards

▶ The diagnosis of depression is clearly communicated in the letter to the referrer.
▶ Clinical notes contain the following information from assessment:
  ▷ comorbid conditions
  ▷ family context
  ▷ school context
  ▷ peer relationships.

Psychological treatment standards

▶ A relevant evidence-based treatment modality (e.g. cognitive–behavioural therapy or interpersonal psychotherapy) is clearly documented.
▶ Psychological treatment is reviewed regularly.

Medication treatment standards

▶ Fluoxetine is chosen as the first-line medication for depression.
▶ Medication is monitored regularly (at least monthly in the first 3 months).
▶ There is clear documentation of discussion of the risks and benefits.

The target is that all of the above standards are met.

Method

Data collection

Cases that had been coded on the CAMHS database as moderate or severe depressive disorder were collected. Information was obtained from the following sources: the assessment letter and subsequent letters for the first 3 months, including multidisciplinary review sheets.

Data analysis

The percentage of patients coded with a moderate or severe depressive disorder for whom the above standards were met was calculated.

Resources required

People

Data collection could be carried out by staff at multidisciplinary team meetings. A coordinator is needed to plan the data collection sessions, to design the pro formas and to analyse the data.

Time

It is estimated that for 30 sets of notes, 10 hours will be required for data collection. Another 2–3 hours are required to coordinate the process and analyse the data.

Results

- ▶ Thirty sets of case notes of patients with a current database coding of moderate or severe depression were analysed.
- ▶ The diagnosis was clearly documented in the letter to referrer in 23 cases (77%).
- ▶ A large range of psychological treatments were used, not all evidence based, ranging from supportive counselling to cognitive analytic therapy.
- ▶ Psychological treatment was reviewed regularly in 17 of 27 cases (63%).
- ▶ Fluoxetine was used as a first-line treatment in 15 of 21 cases (71%).
- ▶ Discussion with the family of risks and benefits was documented in 13 of 21 cases (62%).
- ▶ Medication was monitored at least monthly for the first 3 months in 12 of 21 cases (57%).

Recommendations

An assessment and management checklist should be incorporated into the clinical notes of those patients with an identified diagnosis of moderate or severe depression. This could include a checklist of assessment questions (including diagnosis) as well as a tick-box for management standards agreed as important by the multidisciplinary team, in line with NICE guidance.

Goodyer, I., Dubicka, B., Wilkinson, P., et al (2007) Selective serotonin reuptake inhibitors (SSRIs) and routine specialist care with and without cognitive behaviour therapy in adolescents with major depression: randomised controlled trial. BMJ, 335, 142–146.

National Institute for Health and Clinical Excellence (2005) Depression in Children and Young People: Identification and Management in Primary, Community and Secondary Care (CG28). NICE. Available at http://www.nice.org.uk/CG28 (accessed October 2010).

13. Eating disorders: management

Alvina Ali

Setting

This audit would be relevant in eating disorders services, particularly in outpatient settings. It was originally conducted for an eating disorders service within a child and adolescent mental health service (CAMHS), but it would also be appropriate in adult services.

Background

Eating disorders comprise a range of syndromes with physical, psychological and social features. The provision of psychiatric treatment by high-quality, age-appropriate, specialist eating disorder services has a clear effect on patient outcomes. The purpose of this audit was to ensure that the local service provision was in line with national standards.

Standards

According to the 2004 guideline on eating disorders produced by the National Institute for Health and Clinical Excellence (NICE):

▶ most patients with anorexia and bulimia nervosa should be managed on an out-patient basis

▶ psychological therapies should be offered to all patients who are diagnosed with an eating disorder

▶ psychological therapy for anorexia nervosa should last at least 6 months.

The target is that these standards are met for all patients diagnosed with specific eating disorders.

Method

Data collection

Data were collected, using a specific data tool, from all the referrals to an eating disorder service over 1 year. The data tool allowed information to be collected on the following areas:

▶ diagnosis at first assessment

▶ treatment offered (psychological, parent psycho-education, medication) and whether it was delivered on an out-patient or in-patient basis

▶ types of psychological therapy offered (e.g. family therapy, individual psychodynamic therapy, interpersonal therapy, cognitive–behavioural therapy or a combination)

▶ duration of therapy.

Data analysis

The percentage of the sample with documentation of a diagnosis in line with the ICD–10 classification was recorded. In addition, for patients who required treatment, the percentages with documentation of the following were calculated:

- ▶ type of treatment offered (psychological, others, combined)
- ▶ type of psychological therapy offered
- ▶ duration of therapy (recorded as less than or more than 6 months).

Resources required

People

The audit should be undertaken by at least two people, owing to the amount of information collected.

Time

For a service receiving 100 referrals per year it is estimated that the data collection would take around 15 hours.

Results

The documentation of in-patient/out-patient status, type of treatment and treatment duration was generally good. However, there was inconsistency in the documentation of diagnoses other than anorexia nervosa or bulimia nervosa and also the type of psychological therapy offered.

Recommendations

- ▶ A standardised classification system, such as ICD–10 or DSM–IV, should be used to assign a diagnosis, as this would help staff follow the guidance on the treatment of the eating problem.
- ▶ A specific session on how to use ICD–10 codes of classification for all the staff working within the team should be organised.
- ▶ As psychological therapies are the main treatment offered, clear documentation of the type of therapy offered is very important. The targets and duration of treatment should be specified, along with the level of intervention in each case.

National Institute for Health and Clinical Excellence (2004) *Eating Disorders: Core Interventions in the Treatment and Management of Anorexia Nervosa, Bulimia Nervosa and Related Eating Disorders* (CG9). NICE. Available at http://www.nice.org.uk/CG009 (accessed October 2010).

14. Epilepsy: management

Cameron Martin

Setting

This audit was done in relation to out-patients served by four consultant psychiatrists specialising in intellectual disability (ID). The standards of care are the same for a non-ID population, so this audit could be adapted to any population for whom the clinician has a responsibility for managing epilepsy.

Background

Epilepsy is a chronic illness which poses a challenge in the balance between side-effects and effective treatment. It is particularly relevant to an ID population as the prevalence is higher in this group than in the general population. The risks to the individual are high if the wrong balance is struck, leaving the patient either with frequent seizures and the increased risk of sudden unexplained death in epilepsy (SUDEP) or exposed to harmful side-effects.

Standards

The guidance on epilepsy in adults and children produced by the National Institute for Health and Clinical Excellence (NICE) (Stokes *et al*, 2004) presents 17 standards. All these could be audited, but key minimum standards which should be easily addressed through this type of audit would be the following:

▶ The records show that all individuals have had their seizures and/or epilepsy syndrome classified using a multi-axial classification scheme.
▶ The records show that combination anti-epileptic drug therapy, if prescribed, followed an adequate trial of monotherapy.
▶ The records show that all individuals with epilepsy have had a review in the previous 12 months.
▶ The records show that seizure frequency has been documented in the past 12 months.

Method

Data collection

A sample of the departmental case-load was systematically assessed and all cases of epilepsy were identified. Notes were examined in reverse chronological order. In all notes, the following information was sought:

▶ description of seizures (ictal phenomenology)
▶ seizure type
▶ syndrome
▶ aetiology
▶ reference to the number of anti-epileptic drugs taken and, where more than one drug was being taken, documentation of at least two periods of monotherapy that failed to gain adequate results
▶ review of epilepsy at least every 12 months
▶ review of seizure frequency at least every 12 months.

Data analysis

Database software was used to evaluate the proportion of patients meeting the above criteria.

Resources required

People

This audit can be done by a single person or a small group. Ideally, the auditors should be doctors or specialist nurses, owing to the likely complexity of medical terminology in the records.

Time

If there is no readily available list of patients with epilepsy, forming a list through systematic sampling may take considerable extra time. Once the records are available, it takes roughly 5 minutes per record to assess the above information. It is unlikely that more than 20 records per full-time consultant team would be needed, and data entry should take less than an hour for 20 patients.

Results

The use of multi-axial classification was often missed and there was a lack of recording of reasons for not using monotherapy. The majority of patients were seen twice as often as the minimum standard.

Recommendations

The results of the audit should be presented to the team to highlight the importance of recording a diagnosis using a multi-axial classifcation and recording the justification for combination therapy.

There are numerous other standards which can be audited at the same time, such as level of information given about:

▶ side-effects
▶ drug interactions
▶ safety of daily activities
▶ risks in pregnancy
▶ prognosis.

Stokes, T., Shaw, E. J., Juarez-Garcia, A., *et al* (2004) *Clinical Guidelines and Evidence Review for the Epilepsies: Diagnosis and Management in Adults and Children in Primary and Secondary Care*. Royal College of General Practitioners, pp. 81–82. Available at http://www.nice.org.uk/nicemedia/live/10954/29533/29533.pdf (accessed October 2010).

15. Opiate dependence and pregnancy

Rakesh Magon and Christos Kouimtsidis

Setting

This audit is relevant to addiction teams who are involved in treating opiate dependence in pregnancy.

Background

The extent of drug use in pregnancy is underestimated owing to the stigma and secrecy associated with problem drinking and drug use. The Confidential Enquiry into Maternal and Child Health (2007) reported that substance misuse was directly or indirectly related to 57 out of 295 reported deaths (12 of people dependent on alcohol, 45 of people dependent on illicit drugs). The report concluded that more women were dying from the consequences (direct and indirect) of substance misuse than from other psychiatric causes. The majority of them did not get care from integrated drug addiction services or were poorly managed, with significant inter-agency communication failures.

Standards

The standards for this audit were obtained from *Drug Misuse and Dependence: UK Guidelines on Clinical Management* (Department of Health, 2007):

▶ All pregnant mothers who are opiate dependent should receive substitute drugs to achieve stability. Alternatively, detoxification, if preferred by the patient, can be given but only after the first trimester.
▶ Management should involve good inter-agency liaison and care coordination.
▶ The risks and benefits of treatment/medications should be discussed with all patients, and the discussion documented.

Method

Data collection

A time period was chosen that was long enough to allow a reasonable number of pregnancy cases to be examined but short enough to make clarifications required by key workers reliable. Key workers from each addiction team identified women who were pregnant in the audit period. The case notes were then examined to answer the following questions relating to the above standards:

▶ Did the patient receive substitute drugs to achieve stability or detoxification?
▶ If patient received substitute drugs to achieve detoxification, was detoxification done after the first trimester?
▶ Was patient's treatment preference (substitute drugs for stability or detoxification) clearly documented?
▶ Was a risk–benefit analysis of treatment discussed and clearly documented?
▶ Did the management involve good inter-agency liaison in the following domains:
  ▷ correspondence with the general practitioner (GP)

> ▷ liaison with midwives, community mental health teams, housing depart-
> ments and children's, school and family services where appropriate
> ▷ professional meetings with professionals and agencies involved in client's
> care planning
> ▷ services delivered to drug-using partners.

Data analysis

Descriptive statistics were used in the analysis of the results.

Resources required

People

This audit can comfortably be undertaken by one person based on a total case-load in the region of 1000 patients, with 20 identified pregnancy cases.

Time

Data collection takes 20–25 hours.

Results

Substitute drugs or detoxification for all women concurred with the treatment guideline in all cases. Minor but significant gaps in inter-agency liaison were highlighted. Inter-agency liaison with GPs was not done in 10% of cases, with midwives in 24%, with children's, school and family services in 11% and with housing services in 24%. Professional meetings were missing for 33% of clients. Risk–benefit analysis was documented in 67% of cases. One of the addiction teams audited had no gaps in inter-agency liaison. This team had a key worker with a special interest in care for pregnant drug users.

Recommendations

► There should be better liaison and documentation of discussions with antenatal services and all other services involved.

► Assertive management during pregnancy is warranted, along with clear documentation in the case notes of the patient's treatment preference and risk–benefit analysis.

► Team members should be encouraged to develop a specialist interest in the management of pregnant patients.

► Inter-agency and patient communication could be improved through the provision of information leaflets, education and training for staff.

Confidential Enquiry into Maternal and Child Health (2007) *Saving Mothers' Lives: Reviewing Maternal Deaths to Make Motherhood Safer – 2003–2005. The Seventh Report on Confidential Enquiries into Maternal Deaths in the United Kingdom*. CEMACH. Available at http://www.cmace.org.uk/getattachment/26dae364-1fc9-4a29-a6cb-afb3f251f8f7/Saving-Mothers%E2%80%99-Lives-2003-2005-%28Full-report%29.aspx (accessed October 2010).

Department of Health (2007) Pregnancy and neonatal care. In *Drug Misuse and Dependence: UK Guidelines on Clinical Management*, pp. 80–83. DH. Available at http://www.nta.nhs.uk/guidelines-clinical-management.aspx (accessed October 2010).

16. Schizophrenia: family interventions

Vishwanath Byregowda Ramakrishna

Setting

This audit is particularly relevant to general adult and forensic psychiatry, in both in-patient and out-patient settings.

Background

It has been suggested that high levels of expressed emotion (criticism, hostility or over-involvement) in families of individuals with schizophrenia causes more frequent relapses. A Cochrane systematic review (Pharoah *et al*, 2006) suggested that family interventions may decrease the frequency of relapse, reduce hospital admission, encourage compliance with medication and decrease general social impairment. The 2009 guideline on the treatment and management of schizophrenia from the National Institute for Health and Clinical Excellence (NICE) strongly recommends the implementation of family interventions in schizophrenia.

Standards

The following standards are contained in the NICE guideline:
- Family intervention should be offered to all families who live with or who are otherwise in close contact with patients with schizophrenia. This can be started either during the acute phase or later, including in in-patient settings.
- Family intervention should:
  - include the patient if practical
  - include at least 10 planned sessions over a period of 3 months to 1 year
  - take into account any preference for single-family rather than multi-family intervention
  - take into account the relationship between the main carer and the patient
  - have a specific supportive, educational or treatment function
  - include negotiated problem-solving or crisis-management work.

Method

Data collection

A list of all patients with schizophrenia who were discharged within the past year was obtained from the medical records department. The sample size and the study period may need to be locally agreed. About 20 patients over 6–12 months was considered reasonable. Data were collected mainly from patient medical records. The patient's social worker and/or community psychiatric nurse (CPN) provided additional information.

The following were assessed:
- Did the patient have a diagnosis of schizophrenia?
- If so, was the patient living with or in close contact with his/her family?

('Close contact' is not defined in the NICE guidelines and so may have to be locally defined for the purposes of the audit.)

▶ If so, was the family intervention offered by the team and was it accepted or declined? (There should also be an assessment of whether the patient had the capacity to consent.)

▶ If a family intervention was undertaken, what was its nature and duration?

Data analysis

Compliance with standards was calculated as the percentage of patients who were offered family intervention as per the NICE guideline (including those who refused or lacked capacity to consent).

Resources required

People

At least two people are required to review the notes, depending on the sample size and study period. The audit lends itself to multidisciplinary involvement, especially with social workers and CPNs.

Time

At least 1 month should be allowed (longer for a larger sample).

Results

An initial audit was done based on the previous NICE guideline for schizophrenia, which was similar to its updated guideline in relation to family interventions. This was conducted in a medium-secure in-patient setting and revealed that only a minority of patients were offered family interventions and the standards were met in only one instance. Improvements were instituted (see below) and a re-audit was done just over 1 year later. More patients were offered family interventions, but the standards were still not met for all patients.

Recommendations

▶ The NICE guideline should be disseminated to all staff, especially key members of the team who may be involved in facilitating family interventions (e.g. psychiatrists, psychologists, social workers, CPNs).

▶ The offer of family interventions to eligible patients could be formally considered at meetings (under the care programme approach) either soon after admission or at the time of discharge.

▶ Documentation should be improved, especially when the patient or family refuses the offer of a family intervention.

National Institute for Health and Clinical Excellence (2009) *Schizophrenia: Core Interventions in the Treatment and Management of Schizophrenia in Primary and Secondary Care* (CG82). NICE. Available at http://guidance.nice.org.uk/CG82 (accessed October 2010).

Pharoah, F., Mari, J., Rathbone, J., *et al* (2006) Family intervention for schizophrenia. *Cochrane Database of Systematic Reviews*, (4). Available at http://www2.cochrane.org/reviews/en/ab000088.html (accessed October 2010).

17. Schizophrenia: management

Rob Macpherson and Krishen Ranganath

Setting

This audit is likely to be most relevant in general adult psychiatry and out-patients. It could also be applied to rehabilitation and forensic units.

Background

The National Institute for Health and Clinical Excellence (NICE) has published an updated clinical guideline for schizophrenia (National Institute for Health and Clinical Excellence, 2009a), with separate audit support tools for pharmacological interventions, organisational criteria and clinical criteria.

Standards

The NICE 'clinical criteria' audit support tool has 20 criteria (National Institute for Health and Clinical Excellence, 2009b). Although it would be possible to audit against all 20 criteria, in practice this would be difficult, as some relate to specific phases of illness. When auditing longer-term treatment, the following criteria from the audit support tool can be applied:

▶ All patients should receive a comprehensive multidisciplinary assessment, including a psychiatric, psychological and physical health assessment.

▶ Advanced statements should be recorded and copies kept in the primary and secondary care plans.

▶ Service users who wish second opinion should be supported in obtaining one.

▶ Service users should have a crisis plan, with key clinical contacts noted.

▶ Service users should have one-to-one cognitive–behavioural therapy (CBT), over at least 16 sessions, following a treatment manual.

▶ If the service user lives with, or is otherwise in close contact with, his/her family, they should be offered a family intervention.

▶ Counselling or supportive therapy should not be offered unless the individual requests this or CBT is not available locally.

▶ Adherence therapy (as a specific intervention) should not be offered.

▶ Social skills training (as a specific intervention) should not be offered.

▶ The service user should have routine recording of daytime activities in the care plans.

▶ Staff should give the service user written information about schizophrenia, its treatment and the service providing treatment and care.

▶ If there is a carer, and the service user agrees, he/she should be given written information about schizophrenia, its treatment and the service providing the treatment and care.

In all cases the standard should be 100%.

Method

Data collection

A 12-item data-collection tool (modified from the NICE audit tool) was developed. All service users in a team/service with an ICD–10 diagnosis of schizophrenia or schizoaffective disorder were identified. Audit workers carried out a structured interview with each service user's key worker, to ascertain whether interventions had been carried out at any time in the course of the illness. Reasons for interventions not being carried out, such as service user choice or impaired capacity, were identified.

Data analysis
Mostly descriptive data were used. Cross-comparisons of responses to different questions were made through chi-squared tests.

Resources required
People
For a community mental health team (CMHT) with 200 cases, it is likely that fewer than 100 will be patients with schizophrenia and three audit workers could do this work.

Time
An audit of 100 cases could be completed in approximately 15 hours, assuming that audit workers could make appointments for each key worker in turn.

Results
The case-load of an assertive outreach team was audited against the previous NICE guideline and the results were compared with a case-note audit in a CMHT completed 2 years earlier (Macpherson et al, 2008). Rates of compliance with the NICE standards varied from 0% (provision of advance directive) to 85% (written information given). Compliance was greater than in the earlier audit, which was in part due to the problem of information about interventions being difficult to find in the case notes. The method of structured interview of key workers was considered better than reviewing case notes. When refusal, lack of capacity or another indication was taken into account, the NICE guideline was generally adhered to.

Recommendations
- ▶ A training session to raise awareness among the team about advance directives would be useful.
- ▶ Information about interventions should be clearly documented in case notes.

Macpherson, R., Hovey, N., Ranganath, K., et al (2008) NICE guidelines on treating schizophrenia – audit. Psychiatric Bulletin, 32, 75–76.

National Institute for Health and Clinical Excellence (2009a) Schizophrenia: Core Interventions in the Treatment and Management of Schizophrenia in Primary and Secondary Care (CG82). NICE. Available at http://guidance.nice.org.uk/CG82 (accessed October 2010).

National Institute for Health and Clinical Excellence (2009b) Schizophrenia (Update): Audit Support – Clinical Criteria. NICE. Available at http://guidance.nice.org.uk/index.jsp?action=download&o=44550 (accessed October 2010).

18. Schizophrenia: occupational achievements

Lauren Coates

Setting

The most suitable setting for this audit is a service for early intervention in psychosis, although it could be done by any service caring for people with schizophrenia.

Background

Early intervention teams provide assessment and treatment for all first episodes of psychosis for patients aged 14–35 years, many of whom will be completing their education, thinking about further education or seeking employment. The local team has an occupational consultant who links with a partner organisation offering educational and occupational support for people with mental illness or intellectual disability.

Standards

The 2009 guideline for schizophrenia from the National Institute for Health and Clinical Excellence (NICE) set the following standards:

▶ Mental health services should work in partnership with other organisations to enable people with schizophrenia to access local employment and educational resources.

▶ The daytime activities of people with schizophrenia should be routinely recorded, including 'occupational outcomes'.

▶ Early intervention services should offer a full range of interventions, including occupational and educational interventions.

▶ 'Supported employment' programmes should be provided for people with schizophrenia who wish to work. However, they should not be the only work-related activity offered when individuals are unable to work or are unsuccessful in their attempts to find employment.

▶ All service users with schizophrenia, or in this case first-episode psychosis, should be offered an assessment of occupational and/or educational needs and aspirations, and the service should help them to achieve the desired outcome.

Method

Data collection

The service was still fairly new when audited, so it was possible to obtain a list of all patients taken on by the team (a total of 40). Those who had received an assessment with the occupational consultant had a file held at the partner organisation. The initial assessment paperwork was located in these files and contained information on baseline aspirations. For those whose baseline aspirations had been recorded, information was obtained regarding achievements after 6 months and 1 year. For those who did not have a file, the case notes were accessed on the computerised records system to find out whether there was any documentation regarding the reasons for not having had an occupational assessment.

Data analysis

The percentages of patients receiving an assessment and of patients who did not receive an assessment but for whom a reason was documented were calculated. For the standard to be met, all patients should be offered an assessment and there would be a documented reason in all cases where an assessment was not carried out.

Resources required

People

This audit was carried out by one person; however, the patient group was fairly small. If the audit is being performed on a larger patient group, or if paper notes are being used, then two or more people may be required. If working within a team, other team members may wish to be involved.

Time

For a service with 40 patients, data collection would take around 12 hours.

Results

Around half of new patients were offered an assessment, another quarter were already in employment or education, and the remainder were either not offered an assessment or there was no documentation regarding assessment. Of those who did not have an assessment, there was a documented reason in around two-thirds of cases. There was a larger proportion of patients in employment or education after 6 months and several people were still actively applying for jobs. Of the five patients followed up at 1 year, one was at college and two were in voluntary work.

Recommendations

- ▶ In line with NICE guidance, a reminder should be sent to all team members of the importance of documenting both a baseline assessment of occupational and educational status and aspirations, and signposting to relevant services.
- ▶ Occupational and educational assessment should be made a clearly defined part of any initial assessment pro forma or protocol.
- ▶ Training should be made available to all staff to make them aware of the NICE guidance and of local services available for meeting occupational and educational needs.
- ▶ Robust referral pathways are wanted, as are good relationships between mental health services and services offering occupational and educational input.

National Institute for Health and Clinical Excellence (2009) *Schizophrenia: Core Interventions in the Treatment and Management of Schizophrenia in Primary and Secondary Care* (CG82). NICE. Available at http://guidance.nice.org.uk/CG82 (accessed October 2010).

19. Self-harm: assessment

Amelia Orchard

Setting

This audit is relevant to all mental health professionals who assess patients who present with self-harm to accident and emergency (A&E) departments (e.g. liaison workers, home treatment teams and on-call psychiatrists).

Background

Self-harm is a common presentation to A&E departments. All patients presenting thus should receive a comprehensive assessment. This audit was part of a regional audit comparing self-harm assessments in different A&E departments.

Standards

The standards were obtained from a 2004 guideline on self-harm produced by the National Institute for Health and Clinical Excellence (NICE). It states that every person who self-harms and presents to the health service should receive a comprehensive assessment of psychosocial needs and risk by a healthcare professional. As defined in standards 8 and 9 from the guideline, this assessment should include all the following information:

▶ social situation (living arrangements, work, debt)
▶ personal relationships
▶ recent life events and current difficulties
▶ psychiatric history (previous self-harm, drug and alcohol use)
▶ mental state examination
▶ enduring psychological characteristics associated with self-harm
▶ motivation for the act
▶ characteristics of the act (intent, planning, violent methods)
▶ characteristics of the person (hopelessness, forensic history, future suicidal intent)
▶ circumstances of the person (social class, physical illness, social isolation, bereavement).

Any decision to refer for further management must be based upon the combined needs and risk assessment.

Method

Data collection

▶ All self-harm assessments completed by mental health professionals were identified for a certain time period. The records were retrieved from different locations (e.g. liaison notes, A&E notes, home treatment notes).
▶ The hospital used a specific self-harm assessment tool, which made data collection easier.
▶ A data-collection tool was used to determine whether all the relevant information required by NICE had been recorded at each assessment.

Data analysis

The percentage of assessments that had recorded each part of the needs and risk assessment was calculated.

Resources required

People

As this was part of a regional audit, several people were involved at different locations. Approximately two people per hospital are required.

Time

It is estimated that data collection for 50 cases will take 6 hours.

Results

The self-harm assessments included most of the information that was required. This may have been due to the specific self-harm tool used by the hospital. The amount of complete information recorded ranged from 78% for personal relationships to 100% for psychiatric history.

Recommendations

▶ All information from an assessment should be recorded in one place in the clinical notes and all assessments should be stored in one place if possible.

▶ The use of self-harm assessment forms with clearly defined headings makes it easier to include all the information required for the psychosocial assessment.

▶ If any information is unable to be recorded, this should be stated in the notes, together with the reason why.

National Institute for Health and Clinical Excellence (2004) *Self-Harm: The Short Term Physical and Psychological Management and Secondary Prevention of Self-Harm in Primary and Secondary Care* (CG16). NICE. Available at http://www.nice.org.uk/Guidance/CG16 (accessed October 2010).

20. Self-harm: assessment in children

Daniel M. Bennett and Mercedes Acevedo Merino

Setting

This audit is of particular relevance to those services providing assessments to children who self-harm. The original audit was conducted in a child and family psychiatry service covering children up to the age of 13.

Background

The National Institute for Health and Clinical Excellence (NICE) produced a guideline on the topic of self-harm in 2004, with a section relating to the special provision for children and young people. It recommends that all those involved in triage, assessment and treatment should be 'trained to work with children and young people who self-harm' and should be 'adequately trained to assess mental capacity in children of different ages and must understand how issues of capacity and consent apply to this group and have access at all times to specialist advice about these issues'. NICE further recommends that 'All children and young people should normally be admitted into a paediatric ward under the overall care of a paediatrician and assessed fully the following day' and the responsible paediatric team should 'obtain consent for mental health assessment'.

Standards

- ▶ All patients should have a psychosocial assessment.
- ▶ Consent for a mental health assessment should be recorded in the case notes.
- ▶ The assessment should be performed by a clinician trained to work with children and young people.
- ▶ The parents or other responsible adult should be consulted in the process of the assessment.
- ▶ An assessment of risk should be recorded.

Method

Data collection

All patients presenting to accident and emergency (A&E) with self-harm were identified using the department's computer system. The search terms 'self-harm' and 'overdose' were used. The psychiatric case file was then accessed. Where there were no child or adult psychiatry notes, the A&E cards were examined. If they were also unavailable, the children's hospital medical notes were examined. The notes were inspected to determine the following:

- ▶ the nature of the self-harm and age of the patient
- ▶ whether a mental health assessment was requested
- ▶ whether consent for a mental health assessment was recorded by the requesting clinician
- ▶ whether the assessment was conducted by a clinician trained to work with children and young people

▶ whether a risk assessment was recorded

▶ whether the parents or other responsible adults were consulted.

Data analysis

A data-capture tool was used to record whether each case met various aspects of the guideline and a spreadsheet was used for data analysis. The percentage of patients for whom each of the standards (defined above) was met was calculated.

Resources required

People

This audit covers all children presenting with self-harm. The size of the hospital or unit under study will influence the number of investigators required. Two investigators were involved in the data collection and analysis in the original audit, which identified 46 patients presenting 49 episodes. It is necessary to have good links with the paediatric and A&E staff in order to ensure that the recommendations can be implemented successfully.

Time

Using the model described above and assuming that all case notes are available for access it is estimated that the data collection will take 20 minutes per case.

Results

Two groups of patients were identified; the under-fives, with whom accidental ingestion was most likely to be the presenting complaint; and those in the pre-teenage years, among whom overdose and self-cutting were common. Those who had harmed by cutting were less likely to be referred for a mental health assessment. Of those referred, an appropriate assessment by an appropriately trained clinician was performed in almost all cases.

Recommendations

▶ Those presenting with accidental overdose (especially the under-fives) should not be considered to represent cases of self-harm.

▶ These audit findings should be distributed among appropriate staff in all associated departments.

▶ The guidelines should be re-audited.

National Institute for Health and Clinical Excellence (2004) *Self-Harm: The Short Term Physical and Psychological Management and Secondary Prevention of Self-Harm in Primary and Secondary Care* (CG16). NICE. Available at http://www.nice.org.uk/Guidance/CG16 (accessed October 2010).

II. Legislation

Consent to treatment (Scotland)
Consent to treatment and second-opinion approved doctors
Mental Health Act (Scotland)
Seclusion
Section 17 leave
Section 136 assessments
Tribunal reports

21. Consent to treatment (Scotland)

Daniel M. Bennett

Setting

This audit is suitable for all areas of psychiatry where patients are detained under the Mental Health (Care and Treatment) (Scotland) Act 2003. It would also be possible to convert the methodology to other jurisdictions that use similar mental health legislation.

Background

The Mental Health (Care and Treatment) (Scotland) Act 2003 came into force in October 2005. With regard to documentation of consent to treatment, form T2 is required if the patient consents to treatment, and form T3 is used if the patient does not or is unable to consent to treatment. These forms must be completed within 2 months from the time when treatment was first administered under the Act. Form T3 is completed by a designated medical practitioner (DMP) appointed by the Mental Welfare Commission for Scotland. A separate form, T4, is completed if emergency treatment is given under the Act.

Standards

Standards were taken directly from the Mental Health (Care and Treatment) (Scotland) Act 2003. Of particular relevance were the following:

▶ All patients should have a T2/T3 form completed within the specified time.
▶ The medical notes should contain an entry specifying when the Mental Welfare Commission was informed of the need for a T3 form.
▶ All medication given for mental disorder should be authorised with a consent to treatment form.
▶ If the patient is prescribed high-dose antipsychotics, the requirement for monitoring should be recorded on the consent to treatment form.
▶ A label should be attached to the medication prescription to show that a T2 or a T3 form has been completed to authorise the treatment.
▶ The form, or a copy of it, should be kept with the patient's medication prescription.

Method

Data collection

Initially, the population under study was defined. In the original audit, this was all patients detained for more than 2 months in the hospital. It would be possible to limit this to a particular ward or team. A list of detained patients for the defined population was provided by the local medical records department.

The medical notes, and medication prescription, of these patients were inspected to find entries and documentation regarding the following:

▶ the date when the consent to treatment form was required
▶ the date when the Mental Welfare Commission was informed of the need for a DMP to attend to complete a T3 form

- whether all medication for mental disorders given to the patient was authorised by the consent to treatment form
- whether the medication prescription had a label attached to indicate the completion of a consent to treatment form
- where relevant, whether the consent to treatment form specified the need for high-dose antipsychotic monitoring.

Data analysis

The percentage of patients for whom each of the above standards was met was calculated.

Resources required

People

It is estimated two investigators are required to carry out the data collection and analysis.

Time

Using the model described above, it is estimated that the data collection will take 20 minutes per case.

Results

Poor results were obtained in relation to the completion of consent to treatment (T2/T3) forms.

Recommendations

- A timeline could be used after a patient is initially detained to trigger reminders for consent to treatment documentation.
- Staff should ensure that copies of all consent to treatment forms are kept with the medication prescriptions.
- Training about consent to treatment should be part of the induction training for all new staff, and as part of ongoing continuing professional development (CPD).

Mental Health (Care and Treatment) (Scotland) Act 2003. Available at http://www.nes-mha.scot.nhs.uk/ (accessed October 2010).

Scottish Executive (2005) *Mental Health (Care and Treatment) (Scotland) Act 2003 – Code of Practice*. Scottish Executive. Available at http://www.scotland.gov.uk/Publications/2005/08/29100428/04289 (accessed October 2010).

22. Consent to treatment and second-opinion approved doctors

Lucy Bacon and Clare Oakley

Setting

This audit may be particularly relevant in forensic or rehabilitation in-patient services, where a high proportion of patients will be subject to section 58 of the Mental Health Act 1983.

Background

Section 58 applies to people who are detained under the Mental Health Act and allows for medical treatment for those who do not consent or are unable to give their informed consent to treatment. Treatment can be given for 3 months without consent, and without the section 58 requirements. After this 3 month period Section 58 applies.

Standards

Standards were obtained from the Mental Health Act *Code of Practice* (Department of Health, 2008). Of particular relevance were the following:

▶ If the patient consents, the approved clinician should complete a certificate.
▶ A record of the clinician's discussion with the patient, and of the steps taken to confirm that the patient has the capacity to consent, should be made in the patient's notes.
▶ If the patient does not have capacity to consent or does not consent, then the approved clinician must request a visit from a second-opinion approved doctor (SOAD). The treatment proposal must be given to the SOAD before or at the time of the visit.
▶ The SOAD must consult with two statutory consultees before issuing a certificate approving treatment. Those consultees must be:
  ▷ a qualified nurse professionally concerned with the patient's care
  ▷ another person similarly concerned, who has direct knowledge of the patient in a professional capacity, but who is not a nurse, a doctor or the patient's approved or responsible clinician
▶ The consultees should make a record of the consultation with the SOAD, and this should be placed in the patient's records.
▶ The approved clinician must communicate the results of the SOAD visit to the patient.
▶ A copy of the certificate relating to medication should be kept with the patient's medication chart.

The target is that these standards are met for all patients subject to section 58.

Method

Data collection

Hospital managers should ensure a system is in place to determine which patients are subject to section 58. A list of patients currently in hospital subject to section

58 was obtained from the medical records department. The medical notes of these patients were examined to find entries documenting the following:

► discussion with the patient about the treatment
► the capacity and willingness of the patient to consent
► the SOAD request and treatment plan
► consultation by the two statutory consultees
► the approved clinician's communication of the outcome of the SOAD visit to the patient.

In addition, it was noted whether the current section 58 certificate was kept with the patient's medication card.

Data analysis

The percentage was calculated of patients subject to section 58 for whom the following standards were met:

► For all patients:
  ▷ documentation of discussion about treatment
  ▷ documentation of capacity and consent
  ▷ current certificate kept with medication card.
► For patients who required a SOAD:
  ▷ treatment plan recorded
  ▷ documentation of consultation with SOAD by two statutory consultees
  ▷ documentation of clinician communicating the outcome of the SOAD visit to the patient.

Resources required

People

It is suggested that this audit is undertaken by at least two people, owing to the amount of information to be collected.

Time

For a service with 50 patients subject to section 58, half requiring a SOAD, it is estimated that the data collection would take 12 hours.

Results

The documentation of discussions about treatment, capacity and consent was generally good. However, the documentation regarding statutory consultees was poor. After implementing the recommendations below, this had improved dramatically when re-audited 18 months later.

Recommendations

► A memorandum should be sent to all staff in all professions reminding them of their responsibilities under section 58, as outlined in the Code of Practice.
► Consent to treatment should be covered in the induction training for all new staff and be part of ongoing staff training.

Department of Health (2008) Code of Practice: Mental Health Act 1983. The Stationery Office. Available at http://www.dh.gov.uk/en/Publicationsandstatistics/Publications/PublicationsPolicyAndGuidance/DH_084597 (accessed October 2010).

23. Mental Health Act (Scotland)

Daniel M. Bennett and Sumit Sharma

Setting

This audit is suitable for all areas of psychiatry where patients are detained under the Mental Health (Care and Treatment) (Scotland) Act 2003. In the original audit, a general adult psychiatry ward was the setting. It would also be possible to convert the methodology to other jurisdictions that use similar mental health legislation.

Background

The Mental Health (Care and Treatment) (Scotland) Act 2003 came into force in October 2005. It suggests that the short-term detention order is used as a 'gateway order'. It specifies a number of principles that must be considered by any person utilising the provisions of the Act. One of these is that patients should participate in all aspects of their care, treatment and support. Patients are also given the option of preparing an advanced statement, which has to be considered when delivering their care.

Standards

Standards are taken directly from the Mental Health (Care and Treatment) (Scotland) Act 2003. Of particular relevance were the following:

- ▶ In at least two-thirds of admissions involving the Mental Health Act, a short-term detention certificate should be used.
- ▶ All patients should have any subsequent detentions made within the specified period.
- ▶ All section papers should be present in the case notes.
- ▶ All patients should have copies of the relevant detention and letters informing them about their detention and rights.
- ▶ All named persons should receive copies.
- ▶ All documentation of suspension or revocation should be recorded in the case notes.

Method

Data collection

Initially, the population under study was defined. In the original audit, the population included all patients detained in one general adult ward and corresponding community mental health teams (CMHTs) over 1 year. A list of detained patients was kept by the local medical records department. The medical notes were inspected to find the following:

- ▶ the type of detention certificate used at the time of admission
- ▶ the timing of subsequent detentions
- ▶ copies of relevant section papers
- ▶ copies of letters informing the patient of his or her rights

▶ evidence of the named person having been informed and evidence of appropriate copies having been sent to him or her

▶ documentation on the suspension or revocation of detention (if relevant).

Data analysis

The percentage of patients subject to each type of detention was calculated. The percentage of patients for whom each of the standards was met was calculated.

Resources required

People

The original audit was limited to the CMHTs covering one ward for a period of 1 year. It was sufficient for two investigators to be involved in the data collection and analysis.

Time

Using the model described above, it is estimated that the data collection will take 20 minutes per case.

Results

The standard of using the short-term detention was achieved. Section papers were available in most cases but evidence of letters sent was available in fewer cases.

Recommendations

▶ Copies of all section papers should be filed in the appropriate section of the case notes.

▶ Copies of letters, to the relevant parties, regarding rights should be included in the case notes.

Mental Health (Care and Treatment) (Scotland) Act 2003. Available at http://www.nes-mha.scot.nhs.uk/ (accessed October 2010).

Scottish Executive (2005) *Mental Health (Care and Treatment) (Scotland) Act 2003 – Code of Practice*. Scottish Executive. Available at http://www.scotland.gov.uk/Publications/2005/08/29100428/04289 (accessed October 2010).

24. Seclusion

Ratna Ghosh

Setting

This audit may be particularly relevant in adult and forensic in-patient units, where a small but significant number of patients may be subject to restraint and seclusion.

Background

The aim of seclusion is to contain severely disturbed behaviour that is likely to cause harm to others. It is defined in the Mental Health Act *Code of Practice*. The use of seclusion varies widely across institutions.

Standards

Standards were obtained from the Mental Health Act *Code of Practice* (Department of Health, 2008). Of particular relevance were the following:

▶ The decision to use seclusion is made by the doctor or nurse in charge, and a psychiatrist should attend as soon as possible.
▶ A documented report should be made every 15 minutes in the seclusion record.
▶ The patient should be under continuous observation.
▶ The need to continue seclusion should be regularly reviewed.
▶ Contemporaneous records of the seclusion period should be kept in the patient's case notes. These should document the rationale, use of restraint and medication (given as required, or p.r.n.) and subsequent outcome.

The target is that these standards are met for all episodes of seclusion.

Method

Data collection

A list of patients who had undergone seclusion was obtained from the medical records department. It is the duty of hospital managers to keep these records. The medical notes of these patients were examined to find the entries documenting the following:

▶ the reason for seclusion;
▶ use of restraint procedures and medication
▶ subsequent outcome
▶ gender, age, ethnicity, status as defined by the Mental Health Act and primary diagnosis of the patient.

The seclusion record for each episode was identified and examined for the following:

▶ documentation of the start and end time of seclusion, and the duration of seclusion
▶ whether a psychiatrist was informed, and attended, at the start of seclusion
▶ whether the patient was under continuous observation
▶ whether the need to continue seclusion was reviewed every 2 hours by two nurses and every 4 hours by a doctor and a nurse

► where the seclusion was for more than 8 hours continuously, whether the patient was seen by a consultant psychiatrist.

Data analysis

The percentage of patients for whom the above standards are met was calculated. Data analysed included:

► demographic data of patients subject to seclusion
► the percentage of patients subject to restraint procedures
► the percentage of patients given medication
► the Mental Health Act status of patients
► the subsequent outcomes of patients (e.g. transfer to a psychiatric intensive-care unit or low-secure unit, etc.)
► the documentation of reasons for seclusion.

Resources required

People

This audit can be done by a single person.

Time

For an in-patient unit of 50 patients, this work will take about 10 hours.

Results

► One-third of patients were placed under restraint and half were given medication.
► A few patients, mostly young Caucasian males, were repeatedly placed in seclusion.
► The documentation of the available seclusion records met the standards in all but 2 out of 40 cases.
► Half the patients had a functional psychotic illness; the rest were diagnosed with delirium, acute alcohol intoxication and emotionally unstable personality disorder.
► In all cases, seclusion was used to prevent harm to self and/or others.

Recommendations

► Staff should be educated on the importance of note-keeping relating to seclusion, particularly regarding the physical health variables, and the effects of medication administered.
► Psychiatrists and all other members of the multidisciplinary team should receive training on the use of seclusion and associated policies.

Department of Health (2008) *Code of Practice: Mental Health Act 1983*. The Stationery Office. Available at http://www.dh.gov.uk/en/Publicationsandstatistics/Publications/PublicationsPolicyAndGuidance/DH_084597 (accessed October 2010).

25. Section 17 leave

Suraj Shenoy and John Kent

Setting

This audit is relevant to all areas of psychiatry where patients are detained under the Mental Health Act 1983.

Background

Section 17 leave concerns the controlled movement of patients to areas outside of the ward, unit or hospital building. Leave can be either escorted or unescorted by staff. All section 17 leave for in-patients has to be granted by the responsible clinician in accordance with agreed guidelines within the trust, for restricted patients, within the limits of the leave granted by the Ministry of Justice. However, it is important that patients use their section 17 leave as granted, as non-adherence would render them absent without leave (AWOL), which may have serious implications.

Standards

Standards were drawn from chapters 21 and 22 of the Mental Health Act *Code of Practice* (Department of Health, 2008), in addition to Ministry of Justice policy relating to restricted patients (Ministry of Justice, 2008). Of particular relevance were the following:

▶ All patients who use leave should have been officially granted leave.
▶ All episodes of leave should be with the specified number of escorts.
▶ All episodes of leave should be within the stipulated time limits.
▶ The frequency of the episodes of leave should be in accordance with that documented by the responsible clinician and, in the case of restricted patients, by the Ministry of Justice.

Method

Data collection

Records of leave taken, together with section 17 leave forms, were obtained from ward administration staff and reception registers. The clinical notes, which contain section 17 leave care plans and documentation of leave taken, were examined. The following data were collected for every patient:

▶ If the patient had utilised leave, whether they had first officially been granted section 17 leave outside the secure perimeter of the unit.
▶ The leave had been taken by the patient according to the following pre-specified conditions:
  ▷ the number of escorts
  ▷ the frequency of leave
  ▷ any time limits placed upon the leave
  ▷ adherence to conditions set out in the section 17 leave plan.

Data analysis

The outcome measures were expressed as the proportion of the total leave episodes complying with the above standards.

Resources required

People

It is suggested at least two people participate in this audit. The audit would be suitable for multidisciplinary involvement.

Time

It would take two people about 8–10 hours to gather information on a group of 40 patients. The whole audit, from conception to presentation, was completed in 2 normal working weeks.

Results

The audit showed that the unit was successful in ensuring adherence to granted section 17 leave.

Recommendations

- ▶ Instances of non-adherence to the conditions of section 17 leave should be flagged up at relevant forums within the unit, such as at security committee meetings and clinical governance meetings.
- ▶ The results of the audit should be disseminated to nursing staff on the wards, in order to raise awareness of the issues involved.
- ▶ A re-audit should be done in 12 months.

Department of Health (2008) *Code of Practice: Mental Health Act 1983*. The Stationery Office. Available at http://www.dh.gov.uk/en/Publicationsandstatistics/Publications/PublicationsPolicyAndGuidance/DH_084597 (accessed October 2010).

Ministry of Justice (2008) *Guidance for Responsible Medical Officers – Leave of Absence for Patients Subject to Restrictions*. Ministry of Justice. Available at http://webarchive.nationalarchives.gov.uk/+/http://www.homeoffice.gov.uk/documents/leave-guidance-for-patients.pdf (accessed October 2010).

26. Section 136 assessments

Elena Baker-Glenn and Michele Hampson

Setting

This audit is applicable in all areas where detentions under section 136 of the Mental Health Act 1983 are carried out. The audit could be adapted to the legislation of the devolved nations, for example section 118 of the Mental Health (Care and Treatment) (Scotland) Act 2003.

Background

Section 136 of the Mental Health Act is a power that allows police officers to remove a person from a public place to a place of safety if the officer believes that the person is suffering from a mental disorder and is in immediate need of care or control. Police stations have routinely been used as a place of safety in many areas. The Royal College of Psychiatrists (2008) has proposed a national monitoring form for the use of section 136 orders, which has been developed further and has been successfully implemented in three sites and is incorporated in the form used by the Metropolitan Police. The advantage of using the same data-collection form nationally is that it will assist in benchmarking to enable more rapid service improvement.

Standards

Standards were obtained from the Royal College of Psychiatrists' 2008 report on the use of section 136. Of particular relevance were the following:

▶ There should be routine local monitoring of the use of section 136, by a specific group.
▶ A mental healthcare setting should be used as a place of safety wherever possible and police custody should be used for this purpose only in exceptional circumstances.
▶ An ambulance should be used for conveyance from the public place wherever possible.
▶ The approved mental health practitioner should commence the assessment within 3 hours.
▶ The first doctor should be approved under section 12(2) of the Mental Health Act.

Method

Data collection

The national monitoring form was used to ensure that the data for the key standards could be compared at both local and national levels. For every section 136 detention, the monitoring form was completed by the detaining police officers and by either the approved mental health practitioner or an approved section 136 nurse. The national monitoring form that was used is reproduced in Appendix 1 to this book, and includes information on:

▶ the mode of transport to the place of safety

- the location of the place of safety
- the time police remained with healthcare staff in the hospital place of safety
- the time taken for the approved mental health practitioner and doctor(s) to arrive
- whether or not the first doctor was approved under section 12(2) of the Mental Health Act
- the outcome of the assessment, to give a measure of the appropriateness of the use of section 136
- the total time spent in the place of safety, to identify bed-finding and conveyance problems
- whether or not the person was under the influence of drugs or alcohol, had taken an overdose or required medical attention
- whether or not there were any serious untoward incidents in the place of safety.

Data analysis
For each of the main standards audited, the percentage of cases meeting that standard was calculated.

Resources required

People
This audit should ideally involve a section 136 monitoring group and be multi-agency. The monitoring form will need to be completed by the police and either an approved mental health practitioner or staff at the section 136 suite.

Time
The time taken to complete the audit will depend on the number of section 136 assessments during the audit period in the trust where the audit is performed, and on whether or not the data are already collated electronically.

Results
Early results suggest that, in some areas, police stations are used routinely as a place of safety, police vehicles are used as the main method of transport and there is often a delay in the approved mental health practitioner attending.

Recommendations
- Adequate training should be provided for multi-agency staff regarding their responsibilities and powers under section 136 (e.g. patients wrongly placed on section 136, misuse of police custody suites).
- The monitoring form should be adopted at national level and local monitoring groups should regularly review completed forms and take action if the standards are not met.
- All staff should be trained in the completion of the form.

Royal College of Psychiatrists (2008) *Standards on the Use of Section 136 of the Mental Health Act 1983 (2007) (Version for England)* (College Report 149). Royal College of Psychiatrists. Available at http://www.rcpsych.ac.uk/publications/collegereports/cr/cr149.aspx (accessed October 2010).

27. Tribunal reports

Claire Dibben and Golam Khandaker

Setting

This audit is particularly relevant to general adult or old age psychiatry in-patient services where patients are detained under the Mental Health Act 1983. However, it could be modified to cover forensic patients or patients subject to community treatment orders (CTOs) or guardianship.

Background

In November 2008, the mental health review tribunal was abolished and replaced by the First-tier Tribunal (Mental Health) within the Health, Education and Social Care Chamber for Tribunals. This tribunal hears applications and references for people detained under the Mental Health Act (MHA) and it has the power to discharge patients from orders under sections 2, 3, 7 (guardianship), 17A (CTOs) and 37.

Standards

In 2008, the First-tier Tribunal (Mental Health) introduced new guidance for professionals writing reports. The revised standards for the clinician's report listed below were obtained from the relevant *Tribunals Judiciary – Practice Direction* (Ministry of Justice, 2008). The report, which should be signed by the responsible clinician (RC) or countersigned by the RC if not actually prepared by the RC, should give the following general information:

▶ patient's full name
▶ patient's date of birth and age
▶ patient's address
▶ patient's first language
▶ whether an interpreter is required
▶ date of admission
▶ section of MHA under which the patient is detained
▶ name of hospital where detained
▶ name of patient's RC
▶ period spent under care of this RC
▶ name of patient's key worker
▶ details of any existing advance decisions to refuse psychiatric treatment
▶ date of clinician's report for the tribunal.
  The report should cover:
▶ relevant medical history
▶ patient's mental state and behaviour
▶ treatment for mental disorder
▶ previous self-neglect, self-harm, actual threat or harm to others when the patient was mentally unwell
▶ assessment of risk to self and others if the patient should be discharged
▶ management of these outstanding risks

- assessment of the patient's strengths
- if appropriate, the reasons why the patient might be treated in the community under a CTO as an alternative to continued detention in hospital.

Method

Data collection

A list of patients who had a tribunal hearing during the audit period was obtained from the trust's Mental Health Act administrator. The clinician's reports for these patients were found in the medical notes, which were examined using the above standards.

Data analysis

The total number of reports compliant with each standard was obtained and then converted to a percentage of the total number of reports audited.

Resources required

People

Two or more people should conduct the audit, depending on the number of tribunal hearings that take place in the audit period.

Time

A maximum of 30 minutes may be required to audit each report. Data collection for 50 reports conducted by two auditors should take 2 months.

Results

General information about the patient was adequately covered in the reports, apart from patient's first language and the need for an interpreter. Where the report was prepared by a junior doctor, it was not always countersigned by the RC. Most of the reports included patient's history, current mental state, treatment and history of risk. However, the effects of immediate discharge were not always clearly outlined.

Recommendations

- The Mental Health Act administrator should send a copy of the guidelines for writing medical reports to the RC whenever a tribunal hearing is due.
- Local courses on the use of section 12 should incorporate training on tribunals.

Ministry of Justice (2008) *Tribunals Judiciary – Practice Direction, Health Education and Social Care Chamber Mental Health Cases*. The Stationery Office. Available at http://www.mhrt.org.uk/Documents/3nov08/TribunalJudiciaryPracticeDirection HealthEducationandSocialCareChamberMentalHealthCases.pdf (accessed October 2010).

III. Physical health

28. Diabetes: management

Marlene M. Kelbrick and Ayesha Muthu-Veloe

Setting

This audit was conducted in a tertiary specialist secure hospital, and will be particularly relevant in forensic secure and rehabilitation services with long-stay psychiatric in-patients.

Background

People with severe mental illness are at an increased risk of physical health problems and often find it hard to access good-quality care. Patients with schizophrenia in particular have an increased prevalence of type II diabetes compared with the general population.

Standards

Audit standards were based on the 2008 guideline from the National Institute for Health and Clinical Excellence (NICE) for the management of type II diabetes (see also NHS Diabetes, 2009). Key priorities within the guideline were identified and adapted to suit a psychiatric in-patient setting. Of particular relevance were:

▶ structured patient education at the time of diagnosis, with annual reinforcement and review
▶ individualised and ongoing dietary advice from a healthcare professional with specific expertise and competencies in nutrition
▶ setting a target HbA1c (generally 6.5%) –
  ▷ involve the patient in the decision and give encouragement to maintain individual targets
  ▷ offer therapy interventions (lifestyle and medication) to help achieve and maintain target
  ▷ monitor every 2–6 months according to individual needs until stable on unchanging therapy, and every 6 months once the blood glucose level and blood glucose-lowering therapy are stable
▶ self-monitoring to be offered where possible
▶ management of acute changes in plasma glucose control.

The target was for these standards to be met for every patient with diabetes in the form of an individual care plan.

Method

Data collection

The hospital on-site general practice register or physical healthcare register or prescription charts were used to identify patients with type II diabetes. Data collection was from patient records, care plans, hospital-wide risk assessment and management documents, and ward documents, including nursing care plans, drug prescription charts and blood results. Other sources of information included informal interviews with nursing staff and information obtained from medical staff.

Data analysis
The proportion of patients with diabetes for whom the standards were met was calculated.

Resources required

People
Two people were required to conduct this audit in an in-patient service with 548 beds. Some additional assistance was required from nursing staff and other medical colleagues.

Time
Data collection was completed over 2 months, at 2 hours a day, 1 day a week, covering three wards per week. For a service with 25 wards it is estimated that the audit would require a total of 16 hours for data collection.

Results
Although the majority of patients had regular HbA1c and blood glucose monitoring, less than a third had an individual care plan to address their diabetic management and risk. Of those who had a care plan, few included dietary advice and structured education related to diabetes; a fifth included the management of hyperglycaemia, and just under a quarter included the management of hypoglycaemia. There was also a clear need to improve communication between the general practice and the ward-based multidisciplinary teams.

Recommendations
▶ A multidisciplinary diabetic review group should be established.
▶ Staff training sessions should be given on the management of diabetes.
▶ There should be an individual care plan for each diabetic patient.
▶ Individual diabetic care plans should be attached to each patient's drug chart or placed within each patient's health promotion file.
▶ Re-audit should be done in 6–12 months to evaluate changes/improvements in the service, especially in relation to diabetic control and the management of complications

National Institute for Health and Clinical Excellence (2008) *Type II Diabetes: National Clinical Guideline for Management in Primary and Secondary Care (Update)* (CG66). Royal College of Physicians. Available at http://www.nice.org.uk/CG066fullguideline (accessed October 2010).

NHS Diabetes (2009) *NICE and Diabetes: A Summary of Relevant Guidelines*. NHS. Available at http://www.library.nhs.uk/Diabetes/ViewResource.aspx?resID=298281 (accessed October 2010).

Acknowlegements
With special thanks to Dr Marco Picchioni for his advice and support during the project.

29. Infection control

Floriana Coccia

Setting

This audit is appropriate for all psychiatric services but may be more relevant to in-patient units.

Background

Incorporating evidence-based infection prevention and control advice into routine clinical care is believed to be important in reducing the incidence of preventable healthcare-associated infections.

Standards

There are numerous standards relating to infection control to which mental health trusts have an obligation to adhere (including National Institute for Health and Clinical Excellence, 2003; Infection Control Nurses Association, 2005; Department of Health, 2006).

Standards most relevant to the mental health trust can be selected for the audit process. Either single recommendations or combinations can be used. Four domains of care were selected for audit:

▶ *Sharps.* Sharps, needle-stick injuries, bites and splashes involving blood or other body fluids are managed in a way that reduces the risk of injury or infection (26 possible individual standards).

▶ *Hand hygiene.* Hands will be decontaminated correctly and in a timely manner using a cleansing agent, to reduce risk of cross-infection (25 possible individual standards).

▶ *Personal protective equipment.* Personal protective equipment is available and is used appropriately to reduce the risk of cross-infection (21 possible individual standards).

▶ *Specimen handling.* Specimens are handled in a way that negates the risk of cross-infection to all staff (18 possible individual standards).

The standards should be met in all areas in all domains.

Method

Data collection

The data related largely to the presence or absence of equipment on the ward. A tick-box data-collection sheet covering all relevant domains was used. This sheet contained the four main domain headings and the individual standards within each domain. For each standard the auditor indicated whether the standard was met (Yes/No/Not applicable).

Data analysis

Data were collated using spreadsheet software. Compliance with the standards was calculated for:

▶ the four domains described in the standards above

▶ the individual standards within each domain
▶ each trust, locality or team.

Resources required

People

This audit was coordinated by an audit facilitator; at each site at least one person collected data.

Time

Each individual required at least 1 hour to collect the data on the local ward or unit, but this depends on the size of the unit.

Results

There was a low return rate (47%) and some of the standards were felt to be irrelevant at some sites. There was good compliance with the 'sharps' standards, but other domains required greater staff awareness.

Recommendations

▶ The results of the audit should be sent to clinical staff.
▶ The audit tool should be modified and improved, with staff consultation, to make it more relevant to local areas.
▶ Access to clinical washbasins needs to be improved (more of them should be installed).

Department of Health (2006) *Essential Steps to Safe, Clean Care: Reducing Healthcare-Associated Infection*. The Stationery Office. Available at http://www.dh.gov.uk/en/Publicationsandstatistics/Publications/PublicationsPolicyAndGuidance/DH_4136212 (accessed October 2010).

Infection Control Nurses Association (2005) *Audit Tools for Monitoring Infection Control Guidelines Within the Community Setting*. Available at http://www.ips.uk.net/icna/Admin/uploads/AuditTools2005.pdf (accessed October 2010).

National Institute for Health and Clinical Excellence (2003) *Infection Control: Prevention of Healthcare-Associated Infection in Primary and Community Care* (CG2). NICE. Available at http://www.nice.org.uk/guidance/CG2 (accessed October 2010).

30. Metabolic side-effects of antipsychotics

Rohit Bhardwaj

Setting

This audit is of most relevance to assertive outreach teams, where many patients are on long-term antipsychotic medication. It may also be relevant in forensic mental health settings and first-episode psychosis services.

Background

The metabolic syndrome comprises a cluster of features: hypertension, central obesity, glucose intolerance/insulin resistance and dyslipidaemia. These features are predictive of both type II diabetes and cardiovascular disease. There is increasing concern that antipsychotic medications, particularly atypical drugs, contribute to the risk of metabolic syndrome (Allison *et al*, 1999; Taylor & McAskill, 2000).

Standards

The following standards were obtained from the Prescribing Observatory of Mental Health (POMH) (Barnes *et al*, 2008). All patients prescribed or continuing antipsychotic medication should have the following parameters measured at least once a year:

▶ blood pressure
▶ body mass index (or other measure of obesity)
▶ blood glucose (or HbA1c)
▶ lipid profile.

Method

Data collection

Demographic and clinical variables and metabolic side-effect screening data were collected from case notes. The following were recorded for each patient:

▶ age, gender, ethnicity and diagnostic grouping
▶ the names of all regular and as required (p.r.n.) antipsychotic drugs currently prescribed and whether or not the total dose exceeds the recommended daily maximum according to the *British National Formulary* (Joint Formulary Committee, 2009)
▶ the names of drugs other than antipsychotics currently prescribed
▶ evidence of screening for hypertension, obesity, raised blood glucose (or HbA1c) level and dyslipidaemia
▶ evidence of a known diagnosis of diabetes, hypertension or abnormal lipid profile
▶ whether risk factors were picked up through mental health screening.

Data analysis

The data were analysed at three levels: national, trust and assertive outreach team.

Resources required

People

This audit required at least one person from each team involved.

Time

Data collection took around 30 minutes per case, but depended on the extent of the case notes.

Results

In the baseline audit, 6% of the total national sample had a documented diagnosis of diabetes, hypertension and dyslipidaemia. Re-audit of case notes found each of the above parameters had increased to 7%. Screening for the metabolic syndrome in people prescribed antipsychotic medication increased considerably over the year of the project.

Recommendations

▶ As part of the POMH-UK annual meeting, local project teams should be invited to attend a feedback and action planning session, to present local findings and share successful strategies.

Allison, D. B., Mentore, J. L., Heo, M., *et al* (1999) Antipsychotic induced weight gain: a comprehensive research synthesis. *American Journal of Psychiatry*, **156**, 1686–1696.

Barnes, T. R. E., Paton, C., Hancock, E., *et al* (2008) Screening for metabolic syndrome in community psychiatric patients prescribed antipsychotics: a quality improvement programme. *Acta Psychiatrica Scandinavica*, **118**, 26–33.

Joint Formulary Committee (2009) *British National Formulary* (58th edition). British Medical Association & Royal Pharmaceutical Society of Great Britain.

Taylor, D. & McAskill, R. (2000) Atypical antipsychotics and weight gain – a systematic review. *Acta Psychiatrica Scandinavica*, **101**, 416–432.

31. Metabolic syndrome

Delphine Coyle and Rob Macpherson

Setting

This audit is likely to be relevant to all psychiatrists and can be carried out in both in-patient and out-patient settings. It may be particularly relevant in general adult psychiatry.

Background

Some psychiatric illnesses tend to predispose patients to metabolic syndrome, which is a cluster of cardiovascular risk factors. In addition, several psychotropic medications have been linked to an elevated risk of metabolic syndrome.

Standards

There are currently no guidelines specific to the metabolic syndrome. The standards set by the International Diabetes Federation (IDF) (2006) were used. According to these, a principal criterion for metabolic syndrome is central obesity, defined in relation to waist circumference, with ethnicity- and gender-specific values. However, if a person's body mass index (BMI) exceeds 30 kg/m², central obesity can be assumed and waist circumference does not need to be measured. Two of the following criteria also need to be met:

▶ raised triglyceride levels (over 1.7 mmol/l) or on treatment for this lipid abnormality
▶ reduced high-density lipoprotein (HDL) cholesterol levels (under 1.03 mmol/l in males or 1.29 mmol/l in females) or on treatment for this lipid abnormality
▶ raised blood pressure (systolic over 130 mmHg or diastolic over 85 mmHg) or on treatment for previously diagnosed hypertension
▶ raised fasting plasma glucose levels (over 5.6 mmol/l) or previously diagnosed type II diabetes.

The IDF states that once a diagnosis of metabolic syndrome has been made, patients should undergo a full cardiovascular risk assessment, including smoking status, in conjunction with the following:

▶ *primary intervention* – healthy lifestyle, with moderate calorie restriction (to achieve 5–10% loss of body weight in the first year) and change in diet, and moderate increase in physical activity
▶ *secondary intervention* – drug therapy, if required by people for whom lifestyle change is not enough, and who are considered to be at high risk for cardiovascular disease.

The target is that these interventions apply to all patients who meet the criteria for diagnosis.

Method

Data collection

The medical notes of all patients in the service were examined for documentation of the following parameters:

- waist circumference in centimetres
- blood pressure
- fasting blood tests (triglyceride, HDL cholesterol and glucose levels)
- psychiatric and medical diagnoses
- all current medication.

Data analysis

The percentage of patients who already had the five diagnostic criteria measured and available was calculated. The percentage of patients who met the diagnostic criteria for metabolic syndrome was calculated and then re-calculated after any missing information was obtained.

Resources required

People

Owing to the amount of information collected, two people undertook this audit. It is also suitable for multidisciplinary involvement.

Time

Ten hours was required to collect data from 30 cases.

Results

- The documentation of waist circumference was generally good.
- Documentation of blood pressure was excellent.
- Fasting blood tests of triglyceride, HDL cholesterol and glucose levels were documented for just under half the patients.
- After missing information was obtained, it was found that 58% of the patients had metabolic syndrome; 32% of patients were one criterion short of metabolic syndrome.

Recommendations

- The findings of the audit should be circulated and the importance of physical monitoring emphasised to medical staff.
- All patients with metabolic syndrome should be referred to their general practitioner for appropriate treatment.

International Diabetes Federation (2006) *The IDF Consensus Worldwide Definition of the Metabolic Syndrome*. IDF. Available at http://www.idf.org/metabolic_syndrome (accessed October 2010).

32. Monitoring growth and blood pressure in children with ADHD

Chris Pell

Setting

The audit is of particular relevance to services that manage the treatment of attention-deficit hyperactivity disorder (ADHD) in young people and which specifically use both stimulant and non-stimulant medications.

Background

The medication used to treat the symptoms of ADHD can suppress appetite and so affect the growth rate of children. It can also lead to tachycardia and raised blood pressure, both of which may affect the tolerability of the medication.

Standards

Standards were obtained from two sources, the Scottish Intercollegiate Guidelines Network (SIGN) (2009) and the National Institute for Health and Clinical Excellence (NICE) (2008). The former states that:

▶ Psychostimulants should be considered as the first line of drug treatment for the core symptoms of confirmed ADHD/hyperkinetic disorder.

▶ Once an effective dose has been determined, regular review continues to be important, for checks of behavioural rating and side-effects, along with checks of height, weight and blood pressure.

The NICE standards state that, for people taking methylphenidate, atomoxetine or dexamfetamine:

▶ Height should be measured every 6 months in children and young people.

▶ Weight should be measured 3 and 6 months after drug treatment has started and every 6 months thereafter in children, young people and adults.

▶ Height and weight in children and young people should be plotted on a growth chart and reviewed by the healthcare professional responsible for treatment.

▶ Heart rate and blood pressure should be monitored and recorded on a centile chart before and after each dose change and routinely every 3 months.

Method

Data collection

All case files for children in the service with a diagnosis of ADHD were located. A random sample was selected, and information collected using a pro forma. The medical notes of the selected ADHD patients were examined for documentation of the following:

▶ demographic data including age, gender and consultant

▶ whether the child has been prescribed medication for ADHD

▶ whether the child has been reviewed at clinic

▶ presence of updated growth chart in the notes

▶ recordings of heart rate and blood pressure.

The desired standard is that all children prescribed medication for ADHD should have all of this information recorded every 6 months.

Data analysis

Information was processed to describe the age and gender distribution and the number of children managed by each consultant team. The percentages of children were calculated for:

▶ those prescribed each type of medication
▶ those with a growth chart
▶ those seen in the past 6 months
▶ those whose height and weight had been plotted in past 6 months
▶ those whose blood pressure and pulse rate had been monitored in the past 6 months.

Resources required

People

The audit was carried out by one person.

Time

Data collection took four afternoons, mostly taken up with identifying case files of children with ADHD and recording the data for the selected sample.

Results

The majority of children had been seen within the past 6 months and almost all had a growth chart in their case file. Height, weight, blood pressure and pulse rate were generally well documented.

Recommendations

▶ Awareness of the need for monitoring could be increased by a presentation to a local departmental forum.
▶ Measuring equipment should be available within the department.
▶ Growth charts should be routinely placed within new case files as they are made up.

National Institute for Health and Clinical Excellence (2008) *Attention Deficit Hyperactivity Disorder: Diagnosis and Management of ADHD in Children, Young People and Adults* (CG72). NICE. Available at http://guidance.nice.org.uk/CG72 (accessed October 2010).

Scottish Intercollegiate Guidelines Network (2009) *Attention Deficit and Hyperkinetic Disorders in Children and Young People* (Guideline 112). SIGN. Available at http://www.sign.ac.uk/pdf/sign112.pdf (accessed October 2010).

33. Physical examinations: equipment

Hitesh Joshi, Richard Nixon and Katherine Murphy

Setting

This audit is relevant to all areas of psychiatry where physical aspects of health are monitored. It is of most relevance to in-patient units and day hospitals, where physical monitoring is performed regularly.

Background

Physical examination and physical health monitoring are essential to all patients in psychiatry. Guidance from both the National Institute for Health and Clinical Excellence (NICE) (2006, 2007) and the Royal College of Psychiatrists (2009) emphasises the need for physical examination of mental health service users. A range of equipment is required for clinicians to comply with these recommendations.

Standards

Standards were obtained from *Physical Health in Mental Health: Final Report of a Scoping Group* (Royal College of Psychiatrists, 2009). Standards are that the items listed below should be both present in treatment rooms and in working order:

▶ alcometer
▶ auroscope
▶ disposable gloves
▶ examination couch
▶ height measure
▶ neurological testing pins
▶ ophthalmoscope
▶ pulse oximeter
▶ Snellen chart
▶ sphygmomanometer
▶ stethoscope
▶ tendon hammer
▶ thermometer
▶ tuning fork (256 Hz)
▶ urinalysis kit
▶ videocamera (intellectual disability units only)
▶ weighing scales.

The target was that these standards were met for all treatment rooms.

Method

Data collection

Data were collected using a pro forma that covered the items listed above. One pro forma was completed for each area (e.g. a ward treatment room).

Data analysis

The percentage of equipment present in each treatment rooms and in working order was then calculated.

Resources required

People

This audit was completed by two people.

Time

Fifteen minutes was required to audit each treatment room.

Results

None of the areas assessed reached the 100% target set by the Royal College of Psychiatrists' guideline. The following pieces of equipment were often not present or not in working order:

- ▶ auroscope
- ▶ neurological testing pins
- ▶ ophthalmoscope
- ▶ pulse oximeter
- ▶ tuning folk
- ▶ Snellen chart.

Recommendations

- ▶ An identified lead should be chosen on each ward to ensure medical equipment is present and functioning.
- ▶ A specific trolley containing essential blood-taking and physical examination equipment should be stored in each treatment room.
- ▶ A functional auroscope and ophthalmoscope should be available and kept in a specific secure location.

National Institute for Health and Clinical Excellence (2006) *Nutrition Support in Adults: Oral Nutrition Support, Enteral Tube Feeding and Parenteral Nutrition* (CG32). NICE. Available at http://guidance.nice.org.uk/CG32 (accessed October 2010).

National Institute for Health and Clinical Excellence (2007) *Obesity: The Prevention, Identification, Assessment and Management of Overweight and Obesity in Adults and Children* (CG43). NICE. Available at http://www.nice.org.uk/CG043 (accessed October 2010).

Royal College of Psychiatrists (2009) *Physical Health in Mental Health: Final Report of a Scoping Group* (Occasional Paper 67). Royal College of Psychiatrists. Available at http://www.rcpsych.ac.uk/files/pdfversion/OP67.pdf (accessed October 2010).

34. Physical health of in-patients: assessment

Felicity Richards and Floriana Coccia

Setting

This audit is relevant to all psychiatric specialties. It is of particular relevance to junior members of staff, who complete the majority of admission histories and physical examinations.

Background

People with mental health needs are at increased risk of physical illness, morbidity and mortality compared with the general population (Garden, 2005). Many medications used in psychiatry contribute to illness, compounding poor lifestyle choices and socioeconomic difficulties. Admission to hospital provides an opportunity to assess a patient's health status and to start treatment or refer to other specialties if appropriate.

Standards

Standards were obtained from the Worcestershire Mental Health Partnership NHS Trust (2003) guideline on physical health for in-patients. Mental health trusts should have auditable physical health standards. The Worcestershire standards are in line with guidance from the Royal College of Psychiatrists (2009), which also has auditable standards. Of particular relevance are the following standards:

▶ All patients should have a physical examination within 24 hours of admission. If the patient is confused, the examination should be conducted immediately. If the examination is delayed, a valid reason should be documented.

▶ A medical history should be present in the notes, covering past and present illness, family history of physical health and current medication.

▶ A comprehensive physical examination should be performed, including cardiovascular, gastrointestinal, respiratory, genitourinary, neurological and dental assessment, plus height, weight and waist measurements.

▶ The history should include an assessment of risk factors contributing to physical illness, including alcohol and illicit substance use, exercise, diet and sexual health. Physical health screening should be noted.

▶ Clinical investigations should include: urine drug screen, urea and electrolytes, liver function test, full blood count, glucose, thyroid function test and other hormones if required. Documentation of consideration of other investigations, for example radiography, computerised tomography, bone scans and electrocardiography should be made.

Method

Data collection

A sample of 30 case notes from a range of wards was selected to audit over a specified time frame. The clinical notes of the patients most recently admitted to the wards were examined to find evidence of the following:

91

- physical examination within 24 hours of admission, with reasons for delays documented
- confused patient having been examined immediately
- medical history recorded, including past and present illness, family history and medications
- physical examination recorded, including examination of all relevant body systems, dental care, height, weight and waist circumference
- risk factors recorded, including alcohol, smoking, illicit drugs, exercise/diet, and sexual health, plus health screening
- evidence of appropriate investigations – haematology, biochemistry, thyroid function and serum glucose, as well as appropriate further investigations (e.g. computerised tomography), with relevant documentation of results.

Data analysis
The percentage of sets of clinical case notes with the above evidence documented was calculated.

Resources required
People
Depending on the number of wards and/or specialties involved, at least two people will be required to complete this audit.

Time
Six hours was necessary to review and collate information from 30 sets of in-patient notes.

Results
Documentation of physical healthcare and screening fell below the required standards.

Recommendations
- A refresher lecture on psychiatric history and physical health examination should be included in the trust induction. Training should be repeated at the start of rotation dates of junior doctors.
- Appropriate equipment should be available on the wards to allow thorough examinations.

Garden, G. (2005) Physical examination in psychiatric practice. *Advances in Psychiatric Treatment*, 11, 142–149.

Royal College of Psychiatrists (2009) *Physical Health in Mental Health: Final Report of a Scoping Group* (Occasional Paper 67). Royal College of Psychiatrists. Available at http://www.rcpsych.ac.uk/files/pdfversion/OP67.pdf (accessed October 2010).

Worcestershire Mental Health Partnership NHS Trust (2003) *Physical Healthcare Standards: Minimum Standard for All Inpatient Services and Home Treatment Regarding Physical Examination and Assessment for Patients.* WMHPT. Available at http://www.worcestershirehealth.nhs.uk/Internet_Library/wmhpt/061206%20Minimum%20standard%20for%20all%20 inpatient%20services.pdf (accessed October 2010).

35. Physical health of in-patients: record-keeping

Neel Halder and Shoba Salanki

Setting

This audit was conducted in an in-patient intellectual disability service but is relevant to all psychiatrists working with in-patients.

Background

A comprehensive, systematic investigation of physical health is a core component of the psychiatric assessment. If a patient's stay at an assessment and treatment facility becomes prolonged, it is essential that psychiatrists recognise the need for active health promotion, including formal health checks. This is particularly important in the continuing healthcare setting, where psychiatric services, in effect, assume the role normally carried out by the primary care team.

Standards

Standards were obtained from the Royal College of Psychiatrists' 2009 report *Physical Health in Mental Health*. Of particular relevance were:

▶ physical examination of the patient within 24 hours of admission should be recorded in the patient's medical record (where this cannot be done, there should be a clear entry in the notes with an appropriate explanation)
▶ a record of health promotion/screening (e.g. smoking cessation) should be in the patient's notes
▶ medical history should be obtained within 1 week and made available in the patient's notes
▶ for those with epilepsy, a record of information concerning seizure type, frequency and rescue medication should be obtained within 1 week of admission and made available in the patient's notes
▶ weight and blood pressure should be recorded monthly.

Method

Data collection

Information pertaining to all of the above standards should be documented in the patients' medical records. An anonymous pro forma was designed, with a simple checklist corresponding to the above standards.

Data analysis

The proportion of patient records in compliance with the standards was calculated.

Resources required

People

This audit was undertaken by one person. For more than 25 patients, it is advisable that at least two people are involved. It is suitable for multidisciplinary involvement.

Time

Approximately 30 minutes per set of case notes was required. The time taken will depend on the quality of note-keeping and ease of finding the information.

Results

▶ Most patients received a physical examination by a doctor within 24 hours of admission. However, when this was not possible (perhaps because of the patient's extreme agitation), the reason was not adequately documented.

▶ For patients with epilepsy, there was reasonable recording in the notes of seizure type and frequency, but not of rescue medication.

▶ The recording of weight was erratic.

▶ A minority of patients were having their weight and blood pressure recorded as frequently as is recommended in the audit standards.

Recommendations

▶ There should be training opportunities for staff who are involved in performing and recording the data.

▶ Admitting doctors should be reminded of the importance of documenting the reasons why a physical health check cannot be carried out.

▶ A monthly weight and blood pressure chart should be developed to ensure routine measurement of all patients.

Royal College of Psychiatrists (2009) *Physical Health in Mental Health: Final Report of a Scoping Group* (Occasional Paper 67). Royal College of Psychiatrists. Available at http://www.rcpsych.ac.uk/files/pdfversion/OP67.pdf (accessed October 2010).

36. Physical health of patients with severe mental illness

Kamini Vasudev

Setting

This audit is relevant to all psychiatrists but especially to out-patient settings. It was originally done in a service for early intervention in psychosis, but it is applicable to community mental health teams as well.

Background

People with schizophrenia and bipolar disorder have a high rate of physical health problems. The guideline on schizophrenia produced by the National Institute for Health and Clinical Excellence (NICE) (2009) recommends regular monitoring of the physical health of patients (and a similar recommendation is made in the NICE guideline on bipolar disorder – National Institute for Health and Clinical Excellence, 2006).

Standards

NICE recommends the following:

▶ General practitioners and other primary healthcare professionals should monitor the physical health of people with schizophrenia at least once a year.

▶ A copy of the results should be sent to the care coordinator and/or psychiatrist, and filed in the secondary care notes.

▶ As part of the care programme approach (CPA), healthcare professionals in secondary care should ensure that the regular physical health checks are being carried out in primary care.

According to the Maudsley prescribing guidelines (Taylor *et al*, 2007), patients on psychotropic medications need regular monitoring of various parameters, depending upon the individual psychotropic agent, including:

▶ weight

▶ blood pressure

▶ blood sugar and lipid levels

▶ electrocardiogram (ECG)

▶ full blood count, urea and serum electrolytes, liver function tests and prolactin levels.

On the basis of the above recommendations, the following standards were set:

▶ All patients should have undergone at least one physical health check in the previous year.

▶ All patients should have a record of the results of a physical health check in their notes.

▶ An up-to-date report on all relevant physical health parameters should be available.

Method

Data collection

The medical notes of all the patients were examined for the following:

▶ documentation of a physical health check in the previous year
▶ documentation of measured physical health parameters.

Data analysis

The percentage of patients for whom following standards were met was calculated:

▶ at least one physical health check in the previous year
▶ a record of the results of the physical health check in the notes
▶ documentation of measurement of each individual physical health parameter.

Resources required

People

This audit was facilitated by multidisciplinary team involvement.

Time

For a service with 70 patients, the data collection took 12 hours.

Results

At baseline, the audit did not proceed beyond the first standard of recording physical health checks, as so few patients had a health check recorded. The standards were re-audited following team education, when significant improvement was observed on all three standards.

Recommendations

▶ Awareness of the importance of monitoring the physical health of people with severe mental illness should be increased, by holding an in-house workshop and by discussion with care coordinators.
▶ Liaison between primary and secondary care should be improved, especially regarding which parameters to measure annually.

National Institute for Health and Clinical Excellence (2006) *Bipolar Disorder: The Management of Bipolar Disorder in Adults, Children and Adolescents, in Primary and Secondary Care* (CG38). NICE. Available at http://guidance.nice.org.uk/CG38 (accessed October 2010).

National Institute for Health and Clinical Excellence (2009) *Schizophrenia: Core Interventions in the Treatment and Management of Schizophrenia in Primary and Secondary Care* (CG82). NICE. Available at http://guidance.nice.org.uk/CG82 (accessed October 2010).

Taylor, D., Paton, C. & Kerwin, R. (2007) *The Maudsley Prescribing Guidelines* (9th edition). Informa Healthcare.

37. Screening for blood-borne viruses

Meinou Simmons

Setting

This audit may be particularly relevant to substance misuse services, where a high proportion of patients are intravenous drug users (IVDUs). It can be conducted in both out-patient and in-patient services, but may be better suited to the former.

Background

It is important that patients at high risk of becoming infected with a blood-borne viruses (BBV) are regularly screened, for both treatment and infection control purposes. This has been highlighted by the National Institute for Health and Clinical Excellence (NICE) (2007).

Standards

Standards were obtained from the NICE 2007 guideline on opioid detoxification. Two standards were of particular relevance. First, at the start of contact with all IVDUs (i.e. who are new to the service) and for all IVDUs who are known to the service and have a risk history since last contact, there should be a documented discussion with the patient about testing for the following BBVs and, second, a test should be carried out for them:

- hepatitis B
- hepatitis C
- HIV.

The targets are that these standards are met in all patients in a substance misuse service.

Method

Data collection

Service administrators accessed a list of all new referrals to the service each month. This list was used as a basis to track case notes of new referrals. Data were collected over 3 months. The medical notes of these patients were examined to find entries documenting the following:

- discussion with the patient about testing for BBVs
- documentation that testing was carried out for BBVs.

Data analysis

The percentage of patients for whom the following standards were met was calculated:

- For all new referrals to the service in the 3-month period:
  - documentation of discussion about each BBV
  - documentation of testing for each BBV.
- For all IVDUs referred to the service in the 3-month period:
  - documentation of discussion about each BBV
  - documentation of testing for each BBV.

Resources required

People

The audit was undertaken by one person.

Time

Approximately 10 hours was required to collect data from 20–30 new referrals in a month.

Results

The documentation of discussions about testing was generally good, as there was a relevant prompt for discussion in the service assessment pro forma. Conversely, documentation of actual testing was poor, as responsibility for follow-up and documentation of results was not clearly designated within the service.

Recommendations

▶ A memorandum should be sent to all staff in all professions reminding them of their responsibilities for ensuring that all high-risk patients are offered screening.

▶ 'Testing of BBVs carried out' after 'discussion of screening' should be incorporated within the assessment pro forma.

▶ Training on the importance of testing for BBVs should be provided to all staff in substance misuse services. This should include treatment options and implications of virus spread to others.

National Institute for Health and Clinical Excellence (2007) *Guidance on Drug and Alcohol: Opioid Detoxification* (CG52). NICE. Available at http://www.nice.org.uk/nicemedia/pdf/CG52NICEGuideline.pdf (accessed October 2010).

38. Screening for breast and cervical cancer

Sofia Jaffer

Setting

This audit is relevant to all female patients over 25 years of age in any hospital. It will be particularly relevant in long-stay wards, such as forensic settings.

Background

Women with mental health problems may be at increased risk for developing breast and cervical cancer (Miller *et al*, 2007), probably because of their under-utilisation of preventative services, decreased access to treatment, effects of mental illness and its treatment on the development of cancer, and risk factors common to both mental illness and cancer (Follette & Cummings, 1967; Xiong *et al*, 2008).

Standards

Routine screening methods are recommended by the Department of Health (2007) to detect breast cancer and to identify cervical pathology in preventing cervical cancer. The screening programmes for cervical and breast cancer run by the National Health Service (NHS) have a target standard of 100% (National Institute for Health and Clinical Excellence, 2003). The NHS breast screening programme provides free breast screening every 3 years for all women in the UK aged 50–70 (50–64 in Northern Ireland). Women between the ages of 25 and 64 are eligible for free cervical screening (25–49 years, 3 yearly; 50–64 years, 5 yearly).

Method

Data collection

All female patients aged over 25 years currently admitted to a medium-secure unit were considered for inclusion in the audit. Patients under 25 years were excluded as they were not eligible for screening for either breast cancer or cervical cancer. Information regarding the patient's age, duration of stay and cervical and breast cancer screening was collected from the medical records.

Data analysis

Data were analysed using spreadsheet software. The proportions of patients who had been screened were calculated:

▶ cervical screening for those aged 25–49
▶ breast and cervical screening for those aged 50–70

Resources required

People

Three people were involved in undertaking the audit.

Time

It took almost 3 months to complete this audit.

Results

▶ Of the women aged 25–49 years, 30% were not screened for cervical cancer.

▶ Nearly 30% of those aged over 50 were not screened for cervical cancer.

▶ For more than 50% of the women aged over 50, for whom breast cancer screening is essential, it was not done. In one case, a mammogram was done because an abnormality was detected by physical examination.

▶ In a large proportion of cases there was no documentation relating to whether breast or cervical screening had been undertaken.

Recommendations

▶ There is a need for proper documentation of information regarding cervical and breast cancer screening on physical examination forms.

▶ There is a need to educate patients about the importance and benefit of screening.

▶ Relevant health agencies should be notified if screening information about a patient is missing or screening has not been done.

Department of Health (2007) *Cancer Reform Strategy*. DH. Available at http://www.dh.gov.uk/en/Publicationsandstatistics/Publications/PublicationsPolicyAndGuidance/DH_081006 (accessed October 2010).

Follette, W. & Cummings, N. A. (1967) Psychiatric services and medical utilization in a prepaid health plan setting. *Medical Care*, 5, 25–35.

Miller, E., Lasser, K. E. & Becker, A. E. (2007) Breast and cervical cancer screening for women with mental illness: patient and provider perspectives on improving linkages between primary care and mental health. *Archives of Women's Mental Health*, 10, 189–197.

National Institute for Health and Clinical Excellence (2003) *Cervical Cancer – Cervical Screening (Review)*. NICE. Available at http://guidance.nice.org.uk/TA69 (accessed October 2010).

Xiong, G. L., Bermudes, R. A., Torres, S. N., *et al* (2008) Use of cancer-screening services among persons with serious mental illness in Sacramento County. *Psychiatric Services*, 59, 929–932.

39. Smoking cessation

Sarah Wilson

Setting

This audit took place on a general adult treatment ward but would be applicable to in-patient wards across all psychiatric specialties.

Background

It has been recognised for more than 10 years that smoking cessation interventions delivered through the National Health Service (NHS) are a cost-effective way of preserving life and reducing ill-health (West *et al*, 2000). Nicotine replacement therapy has been shown to double cessation rates in placebo-controlled trials (Luty, 2002). In line with smoking bans across the UK (March 2006 in Scotland, April 2007 in Northern Ireland and Wales, and July 2007 in England), most NHS trusts should have policies in place for psychiatric patients who smoke, and offer smoking cessation support as part of a package of care. In Nottingham (where this audit was conducted), training on smoking cessation with information about the health benefits, stages of change and available support as well as training in brief interventions is mandatory for all clinical staff who work within the trust.

Standards

Standards that are relevant to in-patients (in any hospital) were obtained from the updated Royal College of Physicians' guidelines (West *et al*, 2000):

▶ Hospitals should maintain readily accessible records on the current smoking status of patients.
▶ In-patients who smoke should be advised to stop as early as possible in the admission and this should be recorded on a readily accessible form and repeated annually.
▶ Specialist cessation counsellors should provide behavioural support for hospital patients who want help to stop smoking.
▶ Smokers should be encouraged to consider nicotine replacement therapy, where appropriate, and assisted with this.

Method

Data collection

The medical notes, nursing notes and drug charts of all patients under the care of an in-patient ward were examined for documentation of the following:

▶ the patient's smoking status, recorded on admission
▶ type of tobacco and amount smoked
▶ for patients who smoke, any record that smoking cessation has been discussed
▶ for patients who express a wish to stop smoking or to cut down:
  ▷ any offer of behavioural support
  ▷ the prescription of nicotine replacement therapy.

Data analysis

- The percentage of in-patients who were smokers was calculated, with a breakdown of how much they smoke.
- For patients who smoked, the following was calculated:
  - percentage with documented discussions of smoking cessation.
- For smokers who express a wish to stop smoking or to cut down, the following were calculated:
  - percentage offered behavioural support
  - percentage prescribed nicotine replacement therapy.

Resources required

People

This audit was undertaken by two people per in-patient area, which is a minimum owing to the amount of information collected at one point in time.

Time

For an in-patient area with 20 patients, at least half of whom smoke, it is estimated that the data collection would take 8 hours.

Results

- The documentation of smoking status was good, but the specifics of amount and type of tobacco product smoked were more variable.
- Around half the patients had a documented record of smoking cessation being discussed and only two out of 20 patients expressed a wish to stop smoking.
- Of these two, only one was prescribed nicotine replacement therapy. Neither was offered behavioural support.
- One patient started smoking after admission.
- This audit was due to be repeated after 6 months, to allow the steps below to be implemented.

Recommendations

- The documentation of smoking status should be improved.
- Discussion of smoking cessation could be encouraged by introducing a readily accessible form.
- All clinical staff should complete their mandatory training to offer personalised brief interventions to encourage smoking cessation and teach behavioural support to aid this.
- The broader issues of boredom and lack of activities on in-patient wards should be looked at, with a view to provide alternatives to smoking and improve global health through health promotion, education and exercise.

Luty, J. (2002) Nicotine addiction and smoking cessation treatments. *Advances in Psychiatric Treatment*, 8, 42–48.

West, R., McNeill, A. & Raw, M. (2000) Smoking cessation guidelines for health professionals: an update. *Thorax*, 55, 987–999.

40. Testing for illicit drug use

Caroline Fell

Setting

This audit may be relevant to psychiatrists working in acute adult mental health in-patient settings.

Background

A third of the general population has used or is using illicit drugs, but the proportion is higher among 'vulnerable groups' (Health and Social Care Information Centre, 2007). People with mental illness are one such 'vulnerable group'. Screening for drug use among psychiatric patients is safe, easy and effective. It can aid diagnosis and management and help with prognosis of symptoms or stability of mental health. The key issue is to recognise that substance misuse may be contributing to psychiatric problems and that, pragmatically, the two problems may have to be treated concurrently (Lingford-Hughes *et al*, 2004).

Standards

The recommendations produced by the British Association for Psychopharmacology (Lingford-Hughes *et al*, 2004) set the standards for this audit. Of particular relevance were:

▶ The assessment of the psychiatric patient in an in-patient facility must cover substance-induced and substance-related disorders.

▶ In order to help distinguish between severities of substance misuse disorders, a complete substance misuse history should be obtained, together with urine analysis and blood tests if possible.

Method

Data collection

Hospital managers and/or ward clerks hold lists of patient admissions. Clinical notes were obtained for all patients admitted within a defined period. Patient records were searched for documentation of drug history, and documentation of relevant investigations for drug screening.

Data analysis

The number of patients admitted to an in-patient unit with a possible diagnosis of substance-induced and/or substance-related disorder was noted. The percentages of patients who had a drug history taken on admission and who had urine analysis results documented were calculated.

Resources required

People

One person was required to review both the admission notes and the laboratory results.

Time

Collecting data took approximately 5 minutes per patient.

Results

More than half the new admissions did not have an adequate drug history documented. This improved with staff education and discussion. The number of urine drug screens performed was extremely low, but this improved on re-audit following awareness training.

Recommendations

▶ Medical staff should be educated about the need to take comprehensive drug histories and about the value of urine drug screening.

▶ A checklist should be included on the physical examination admission document to indicate whether urine testing is appropriate, and whether consent has been achieved.

▶ Individual urine testing kits should be used on the wards if at all possible, to improve uptake of screening.

Health and Social Care Information Centre (2007) *Statistics on Drug Misuse, England*. HSCIC. Available at http://www.ic.nhs.uk/pubs/drugmisuse07 (accessed October 2010).

Lingford-Hughes, A. R., Welch, S. J. & Nutt, D. J. (2004) Evidence based guidelines for the pharmacological management of substance misuse, addiction and comorbidity: recommendations from the British Association for Psychopharmacology. *Journal of Psychopharmacology*, 18, 293–335.

41. Venepuncture equipment

David Middleton

Setting

This audit is relevant to in-patient settings and can be modified according to local guidelines and patient groups.

Background

Appropriate clinical investigations and blood tests form part of the work-up for many in-patient admissions. In particular, they are used to ascertain the role that medical conditions may play in a patient's presentation. They also serve as baseline investigations for the prescription of psychotropic medication and for monitoring physical parameters thereafter. The availability of venepuncture equipment on psychiatric wards is important in the investigation and treatment of patients on psychiatric wards.

Standards

The following standards were obtained from *Physical Health in Mental Health* (Royal College of Psychiatrists, 2009) and the *Royal Marsden Manual of Clinical Nursing Procedures* (Dougherty & Lister, 2008):

▶ Appropriate physical investigations should be completed during the first week of admission.

▶ The venepuncture equipment listed below must be available and accessible on each ward, maintained in working order:

▷ tray
▷ blood specimen bottles
▷ blood test request forms
▷ tourniquet
▷ alcohol swab
▷ gloves
▷ needle and syringe or vacuum system
▷ adhesive plaster
▷ sharps bin.

The target is that these standards are met for all patients and for all psychiatric wards.

Method

Data collection

The medical notes of patients on a given psychiatric ward were examined to determine whether appropriate physical investigations had been carried out within the recommended time frame.

The clinical rooms of each ward were inspected for the availability of each of the items of equipment required for venepuncture, and whether these items were in working order.

Data analysis

The following were determined for each ward:

▶ the percentage of patients receiving appropriate physical investigations within the recommended time frame

▶ whether all appropriate equipment for venepuncture was available

▶ whether all equipment was in good working order.

Resources required

People

This audit was carried out by a single person, but might require the help of additional people to audit wards on different sites.

Time

Two hours of data collection was required for a ward of 25 patients. The majority of this time was needed to gather information about investigations in the medical notes.

Results

▶ All patients on the psychiatric wards investigated had received appropriate investigations within 1 week of admission.

▶ Most wards had the appropriate equipment for venepuncture.

▶ There were some wards that had equipment that was in poor working order, such as out-of-date blood specimen bottles or full sharps bins.

Recommendations

▶ A copy of the venepuncture equipment requirements should be given to each ward. A member of ward staff could be allocated the tasks of checking ward stock against this list on a weekly basis and of ordering replacement stock.

▶ Re-audit should be carried out after the implementation of relevant recommendations.

Dougherty, L. & Lister, S. (2008) *The Royal Marsden Hospital Manual of Clinical Nursing Procedures* (7th edition). Wiley-Blackwell.

Royal College of Psychiatrists (2009) *Physical Health in Mental Health: Final Report of a Scoping Group* (Occasional Paper 67). Royal College of Psychiatrists. Available at http://www.rcpsych.ac.uk/files/pdfversion/OP67.pdf (accessed October 2010).

IV. Record-keeping

42. Alcohol history

Rebekah Bourne

Setting

This audit was conducted in three general adult psychiatric in-patient units, including a psychiatric intensive-care unit. It would also be suitable for older-adult or forensic in-patient settings.

Background

Research has shown that in general hospitals 20–30% of men and 5–10% of women admitted are 'problem drinkers' (Seppä & Mäkelä, 1993). A higher proportion of alcohol misuse and dependence is found among psychiatric in-patients. Hulse *et al* (2000) found high rates of alcohol dependence among psychiatric in-patients using the AUDIT questionnaire: they found that 60% of men and 40% of women admitted to a general psychiatric unit had a level of alcohol consumption that was harmful or hazardous or were alcohol dependent.

Withdrawal from alcohol is associated with significant morbidity and mortality. Therefore, it is essential to identify patients who are admitted with alcohol dependence early, so they can be appropriately managed.

Standards

At the time of the audit, the trust's handbook for junior doctors did not include an alcohol history as a minimum standard for admission clerking. It was felt that, where possible, an alcohol history should be taken within the first 24 hours of admission. The alcohol history should contain:

▶ quantity of alcohol consumed over a set period (e.g. weekly)
▶ if the patient is taking alcohol daily, an enquiry about the presence of withdrawal symptoms
▶ if symptoms of dependence are recorded, an enquiry about any history of seizures on withdrawal
▶ details of any previous attempts at detoxification (when, where, complications, etc.)

These standards were devised using 'Assessment of the patient with alcohol problems' from the *Oxford Handbook of Psychiatry* (Semple *et al*, 2005).

Method

Data collection

The clinical notes of all in-patients in three hospitals were reviewed. The admission clerking and medical and nursing entries for the first 24 hours following admission were checked for entries regarding alcohol history.

Data analysis

The following information was collected from each set of notes:

▶ gender
▶ ethnicity

▶ date of admission
▶ Mental Health Act status
▶ whether an alcohol history was taken within the first 24 hours.

If an alcohol history was recorded:

▶ whether symptoms of dependence were enquired about
▶ whether alcohol dependence was present
▶ if present, whether appropriate management was initiated.

Resources required

People

It is suggested that this audit is undertaken by at least two people, owing to the amount of information collected and the number of sets of notes to be reviewed.

Time

For three in-patient units with five wards, there were a total of 84 in-patients and 82 sets of patient notes were reviewed. This took two people 3 hours each to collect the data.

Results

▶ Overall, very few patients had alcohol histories recorded during their first 24 hours of admission.
▶ A quarter of those who had alcohol histories recorded were diagnosed with alcohol dependence.
▶ Although a large proportion of those found to be alcohol dependent were prescribed benzodiazepines, none was prescribed thiamine or vitamin B.
▶ A patient's ethnicity seemed to influence whether an alcohol history was recorded at admission. In particular, White British or Irish patients were more likely to have a record of enquiry about alcohol use, but few patients of Asian origin did.

Recommendations

▶ Further training should be given to junior doctors on the importance of taking and recording alcohol histories on admission.
▶ This should be one of the minimum standards for admission clerking in the junior doctor's handbook.
▶ Trust guidelines on the management of alcohol detoxification should be disseminated to all junior doctors.

Hulse, G. K., Roydhouse, R. M., Basso, M. R., et al (2000) Screening for hazardous alcohol use and dependence in psychiatric inpatients using the AUDIT questionnaire. Drug and Alcohol Review, 19, 291–298.

Semple, D., Smyth, R., Burns, J., et al (2005) Oxford Handbook of Psychiatry, pp. 510–511. Oxford University Press.

Seppä, K. & Mäkelä, R. (1993) Heavy drinking in hospital patients. Addiction, 88, 1377–1382.

43. Care plans in community drug and alcohol teams

Elizabeth Tanna and Christos Kouimtsidis

Setting

This audit is relevant to community drug and alcohol teams (CDATs).

Background

For over a decade, care planning has been used in structuring the treatment and management of patients within substance misuse services. The central role of care plans and their use has been set out in guidelines and recommendations from the National Treatment Agency (NTA).

Standards

Standards for this audit were obtained from NTA documents and were as follows:

▶ All patients entering treatment with substance misuse services should have a written care plan.
▶ Patients should be involved in the construction of this care plan.
▶ The care plan should be signed by both key worker and patient.
▶ The care plan should be regularly updated and reviewed (the NTA recommends a review 3 months after the initial care plan and reviews every 3–6 months for subsequent care plans).
▶ Within the care plan, information about the following four domains should be included:
  ▷ drug and alcohol use
  ▷ physical and psychological health
  ▷ criminal involvement and offending
  ▷ social functioning.

Method

Data collection

All cases open to each CDAT at the time of audit were identified according to primary substance of use (illicit drugs or alcohol) and by key worker. Then 10% of each CDAT's cases were selected randomly (using systematic sampling to ensure cases selected were not weighted in favour of any individual key worker). The case notes of the selected cases were examined for the following:

▶ a care plan present in the notes
▶ the care plan signed by both the key worker and patient
▶ the date the care plan was last updated
▶ a clearly identified 'treatment plan' documented in the care plan
▶ all four domains included in the care plan
▶ an 'aim' and 'plan of care' documented in each of the four domains.

Data analysis

After preliminary data analysis, clarification was sought from key workers in a random sample of cases to establish whether domains missed had been considered for that client but not documented or had been omitted entirely.

Resources required

People

This audit can comfortably be undertaken by one person in a CDAT managing around 1000 patients. If more than one professional documents care plans, then they should be involved in data collection.

Time

Based on this size of audit, data collection takes approximately 20–25 hours.

Results

- ▶ Care plans were present for approximately 70% of patients.
- ▶ The majority of care plans had clearly defined aims and treatment plans.
- ▶ The frequency of care plan review was low.
- ▶ Care plans were signed by key workers in only 70% of cases and by patients in only half of cases.
- ▶ Documentation in the four domains was incomplete.

Recommendations

- ▶ A standardised care plan format should be designed that can be used in all CDATs in the trust. This should include the four domains within the 'aims' and 'treatment plan' sections and areas for the signatures of both client and key worker.
- ▶ An automated reminder system for care plan review should be devised and implemented.

National Treatment Agency (2002) *Models of Care Part 2: Full Reference Report.* NTA.
National Treatment Agency (2006) *The Care Planning Practice Guide.* NTA.
National Treatment Agency (2006) *Models of Care for Treatment of Adult Drug Misusers: Update 2006.* NTA.
National Treatment Agency (2006) *NTA Service Users Satisfaction Survey.* NTA.
National Treatment Agency (2006) *Joint Healthcare Commission and NTA Substance Misuse Improvement Review.* NTA.
National Treatment Agency (2007) *Care Planning: A Good Practice Guide.* NTA.
Documents available at http://www.nta.nhs.uk/publications.aspx (accessed October 2010).

44. Care programme approach: home treatment teams

Matthew Impey

Setting

This audit applies to all home treatment teams (HTTs) which use care plans based on the care programme approach (CPA) to guide treatment. By adapting the standards, the documents produced by a community mental health team (CMHT) could be similarly audited.

Background

The CPA process was launched in 1992 to guide more patient-focused mental health provision. The interpretation of how to document care plans varies between services, with some using clearly defined forms and others allowing a less rigid structure. The essence of care planning is to organise service delivery around what the patient needs and wants, and to make sure this is reviewed regularly.

Standards

The expected contents of a CPA care plan are not rigidly defined. The 2006 Department of Health policy booklet suggests that they should:

- identify the interventions and anticipated outcomes
- record all the actions necessary to achieve the agreed goals
- give an estimated time by which the outcomes or goals will be achieved or reviewed
- detail the contributions of all the agencies involved
- include appropriate crisis and contingency plans.

Based on this document, a list of standards was drawn up (to apply in all cases):

- A care plan should be present for all patients.
- Care plans should be completed within 24 hours of admission to the service.
- Care plans should include sections covering:
  - ▷ concerns – what needs to be addressed or changed
  - ▷ aims – the goal of this episode of care
  - ▷ interventions – how these aims are going to be achieved
  - ▷ contact plan – a list of review dates and which staff are allocated.
- A record should be present regarding whether the patient has received a copy of the care plan.

As the patient would already be under the most intensive community treatment service, crisis plans were not considered a necessity.

Method

Data collection

Notes from all admissions to the home treatment service were obtained and care plans extracted. Data were collected for all patients on the case-load at a set point in time.

Data analysis

For each of the above points, recording involved yes/no answers only and data were presented as proportions of the total case-load.

Resources required

People

As the turnover of HTTs tends to be rapid, it is best to collect the data in a single day. This may require two people. Alternatively, collection could be over a longer period of time and require only one participant.

Time

As the audit looks at one document only, data collection can be performed in a short period of time. Collecting data during a night shift is a useful option but is at the discretion of the auditor.

Results

Care plans were present for almost all clients, and 72% were completed within 24 hours. Essential contents were present for 73%, with contact dates recorded most consistently. Delivery of care plans to patients was not recorded for any cases, despite a prompt being present at the end of the electronic form.

The findings were presented to the clinical team. Another audit took place 1 month after this. Unfortunately, the second audit found slightly worse results than the first, although all patients had a care plan and they were completed more promptly. The narrative of care plans had become slightly less structured and fewer essential contents were included, however. This suggests a difficulty with conveying important messages, which will be addressed through team meetings. Considering the fast pace of home treatment, it may not be possible to improve results much beyond the present level.

Recommendations

- ▶ The team members should be encouraged to discuss what contents they consider to be essential in care plans, and to consider using a structured 'concerns, aims and interventions' model if no other method is found.
- ▶ The team should discuss the delivery (and how to record the delivery) of care plans to patients.
- ▶ A record of the delivery of plans should appear in individual electronic entries.

Department of Health (2006) *Effective Care Co-ordination in Mental Health Services: Modernising the Care Programme Approach — A Policy Booklet.* Available at http://www.dh.gov.uk/en/Publicationsandstatistics/Publications/PublicationsPolicyAndGuidance/DH_4009221 (accessed October 2010).

45. Care programme approach: prisons

Muthusamy Natarajan and Jayanth Srinivas

Setting

This audit is relevant to all psychiatric specialties with multidisciplinary mental health teams who interact with prisoners on the care programme approach (CPA).

Background

The CPA is an integral part of providing a safe and effective service for those with mental health problems in prison. Continuity of care from prison to the community is a particular conundrum. Prisoner mental health is an important aspect of healthcare. Singleton *et al* (1998) found that 90% of prisoners had psychiatric morbidity (psychosis, neurosis, personality disorder, or substance misuse problems).

Standards

The aim was to analyse the quality of CPA by multidisciplinary teams in prisons as per the standards set out in *The CPA Handbook* (Care Programme Approach Association, 2009):

▶ comprehensive initial assessment
▶ appointment of a care coordinator
▶ date set for the next CPA review (every 6 months and before release, transfer or discharge)
▶ appropriate focus on risk assessment and management
▶ documented care plan, updated appropriately
▶ a crisis and contingency plan that is 'formulated, updated and circulated'
▶ identification of unmet needs
▶ outcomes reviewed using the HoNOS-secure instrument (the Health of the Nation Outcome Scales for users of secure and forensic services), completed initially, then every 6 months and before discharge)
▶ if CPA is withdrawn, that an appropriate handover (e.g. letter to general practitioner) is undertaken (which could include exchange of information, plans for reviews, support and follow-up, and whom to contact if necessary, for example in the case of relapse).

Method

Data collection

Case files (inmate medical records and prison mental health team files) were selected randomly for analysis to determine whether the national standards were being adhered to. These covered all accepted referrals from the prison mental health team, but only those relating to patients who had been discharged were reviewed.

Data were collected using an appropriately devised audit tool, which listed the national standards. In addition, the following data were obtained:

- dates of referral, acceptance and discharge
- age, gender and ethnicity
- index offence
- sentence type
- diagnostic category.

Data analysis

The number of individuals (on CPA) who met the national standards was determined and the percentage calculated. The results were presented in tabular form and in charts.

Resources required

People

It is suggested that this audit is conducted by at least two people, owing to the amount of information that needs to be analysed. Administrative support would be useful.

Time

Data collection and analysis from approximately 25 sets of notes would take up to 15 hours.

Results

- Overall, practice and documentation of the CPA were good.
- In all cases, a care coordinator was identified and recorded, and an initial assessment completed and sent to the referrer.
- A risk assessment was completed in 96% of cases, and identified risks were addressed in these cases.
- Initial care plan completion and subsequent review were good.
- A needs assessment was completed in 76% of cases and an initial HoNOS-secure completed in 64% of cases.
- Areas for improvement were identified, including handover of CPA and care at discharge from the service.

Recommendations

- The findings of the audit should be disseminated to clinicians and healthcare managers, as well as other relevant agencies (e.g. probation).
- Consideration should be given to the appointment of a CPA coordinator to ensure national standards for CPA are met in all cases.
- Re-audits should be done annually to maintain an improvement.

Care Programme Approach Association (2009) *The CPA Handbook*. CPAA.

Singleton, N., Meltzer, H., Gatward, R., *et al* (1998) *Psychiatric Morbidity among Prisoners in England and Wales*. Office of National Statistics.

46. Care programme approach: secondary care

Afia Ali and Angela Hassiotis

Setting

This audit is relevant to all secondary mental health in-patient and out-patient services, particularly services that have a large number of patients with severe mental illness of high complexity and risk, including patients with mild intellectual disabilities.

Background

The Department of Health (2008) has issued new guidance on the implementation of the care programme approach (CPA). Previous categories of 'standard' and 'enhanced' CPA have been removed. The new CPA applies to patients previously meeting the criteria for 'enhanced CPA' (severe mental disorder of high complexity and risk and receiving support from multiple agencies). It also includes key groups such as those with parenting or caring responsibilities, history of substance misuse and a history of self-harm or violence.

Standards

The standards were based on the Department of Health 2008 guidance:

▶ patients on CPA have support from a designated, named care coordinator
▶ a comprehensive multidisciplinary assessment covers the full range of needs, including assessment of social care needs
▶ a comprehensive formal written care plan covers risk and safety, and includes a contingency and crisis plan
▶ a formal multidisciplinary review is done at least once a year
▶ ongoing need for new CPA support is reviewed
▶ advocacy support is available
▶ carers are identified and offered a carer's assessment.

Method

Data collection

Services should ensure that an up-to-date database is kept of all patients on CPA. The medical notes of these patients were examined. The following were recorded on a structured data-collection form:

▶ the presence of a CPA care plan in the notes for the past 12 months
▶ named care coordinator (and profession) on the care plan
▶ presence of risk assessment and whether it was updated following the previous CPA review
▶ documentation of contingency/crisis plan within the care plan
▶ documentation of social and physical issues in the care plan
▶ whether the next CPA date had been allocated.

In addition to the above, the following could also be examined:

▶ whether there had been a discussion of the need for an advocate

▶ whether a carer's assessment had been offered to the main carer (if applicable).

Finally, for patients with intellectual disabilities, health action plans ought to be provided as part of the health needs assessment.

Data analysis

The percentages of patients achieving the following standards were calculated:

▶ CPA care plan in the notes for the past 12 months
▶ documentation of a named care coordinator
▶ risk assessment in the patient case notes
▶ risk assessment updated in the past 12 months
▶ clear crisis plan documented in the case notes
▶ documentation of key issues – housing, benefits, employment, physical health.

Resources required

People

This audit should be conducted by two people from the multidisciplinary team, particularly if there is a large number of cases. The lead health organisation (e.g. primary care trust or foundation trust) should help with data analysis.

Time

For a service with 30 patients on the CPA, 7.5 hours would be required for data collection (assuming one person collects the data).

Results

A CPA care plan for the past 12 months, documentation of a named care coordinator, a crisis plan and allocation of a date for next CPA review were generally recorded in the notes. Weaknesses related to the completion and updating of risk assessments. The results improved after implementation of the suggestions below in successive annual re-audits (Ali *et al*, 2006).

Recommendations

▶ In-house CPA training should be provided for all new members of staff and CPA should be included in supervision.
▶ There should be 30-day reminders for reviews.
▶ Prompts should be included on CPA forms.
▶ A CPA working group might resolve problems with the CPA process.

Ali, A., Hall, I., Taylor, C., *et al* (2006) Auditing the care programme approach for people with learning disability: a four year audit cycle. *Psychiatric Bulletin*, **30**, 415–418

Department of Health (2008) *Refocusing the Care Programme Approach. Policy and Positive Practice Guidance*. DH. Available at http://www.dh.gov.uk/en/Publicationsandstatistics/Publications/PublicationsPolicyAndGuidance/DH_083647 (accessed October 2010).

47. Confidential waste

Neil Masson

Setting

This audit is relevant to all specialties in psychiatry and in all settings.

Background

Doctors have a duty to keep confidential information about their patients safe and to destroy confidential information in a safe and secure manner. Clinical notes and typed letters are often put into general waste bins instead of being shredded. This can result in sensitive information being viewed by third parties, which may have legal or disciplinary ramifications.

Standards

The Data Protection Act 1998 applies to all organisations that hold personal data on individuals. The seventh principle of the Act concerns unlawful processing and accidental loss of personal data, phrased in the Act as follows: 'Appropriate technical and organisational measures shall be taken against unauthorised or unlawful processing of personal data and against accidental loss or destruction of, or damage to, personal data.' The Act advocates shredding of confidential waste to reduce the risk of confidential information being made public. Compliance with the Act is mandatory: failure to comply can result in legal action and fines. The target in this audit was that no patient-identifiable information should be disposed of as general waste.

Method

Data collection

The waste bins in all rooms in a psychiatry department were checked at the end of each day for a set time period without the knowledge of the staff in that department. If confidential waste was identified, it was categorised as:

▶ 'patient identifiable' waste (i.e. that linked an individual to the department)
▶ 'sensitive' waste (i.e. that linked the individual to the department *and* included sensitive information, such as history, diagnosis and treatment).

Data analysis

The number of 'patient identifiable' and 'sensitive' waste items was counted. A brief description of what form they took and where they were found was recorded.

Resources required

People

This audit can be completed by a single person.

Time

This audit may involve staying behind after work for approximately 30 minutes so that waste bins can be examined at the end of the day. This would be necessary for the duration of the audit timeframe.

Results

Several items of confidential waste were identified during the data-collection period, with a few rooms being responsible for the majority. After implementation of the first suggestion below, the amount of confidential waste reduced significantly.

Recommendations

▶ The results of the audit should be presented to all staff in the department and the importance of the Data Protection Act highlighted.

▶ Large general shredding bins should be placed in a central location that is convenient to all.

▶ Shredder bins should be available in all clinical areas (with application for special funding if necessary).

48. Documentation of the psychiatric history

Abigail Taylor and Floriana Coccia

Setting

This audit is relevant to all specialties and can be conducted in both in-patient and out-patient departments.

Background

The documentation of a full and accurate history during a medical consultation is of utmost importance. There is evidence to suggest that 80% of diagnoses may be made on the basis of history alone (Hampton *et al*, 1975). In psychiatry, it could be argued that the history provides 100% of the diagnosis, if the mental state examination is included as part of the history. Case notes are referred to during legal proceedings; therefore, they need to be a complete and accurate record of consultations, decisions and actions (Osborn *et al*, 2005).

Standards

There are no specific standards from the Royal College of Psychiatrists regarding the content of psychiatric clinical notes. Therefore, a standard was constructed using the *New Oxford Textbook of Psychiatry* (a widely used and respected source). The authors outline the 'perfect' psychiatric history (Cooper & Oates, 2003). All aspects of the history should be documented completely (standard of 100%).

Method

Data collection

The medical notes of a random selection of patients were collected. Between 30 and 40 sets of notes was deemed adequate. Only first consultations were reviewed. A pro forma was developed for this audit that covered 11 main areas of the history (a total of 34 subheadings):

- patient identification (name, age, marital status, occupation, ethnic background, circumstances of referral)
- presenting complaint
- history of presenting complaint
- psychiatric history
- medical history
- family history (parents, siblings, medical history, psychiatric history)
- social history (financial, support structures, living arrangements, hobbies)
- personal history (birth, development, education, occupational history, relationships, children)
- forensic history
- premorbid personality (self-description, habits – drug and alcohol)
- mental state examination (appearance and behaviour, speech, thought form and content, mood and affect, perception, cognition and insight).

Data analysis

Each history was assigned a total score out of 34 (one point for each subheading) on the pro forma, which was expressed as a percentage. All the above should have been present for the standard to be met.

Resources required

People

Ideally two people should perform this audit, for independent assessment of the case notes. The auditor should be of the same discipline as the person recording the history. This audit also requires secretarial support for the collection of notes.

Time

Around 20–30 minutes per person per set of notes should be allowed.

Results

- ▶ Most aspects of the histories were well recorded. The few exceptions were ethnicity, hobbies, financial arrangements, forensic history and occupational history.
- ▶ The mental state examination was fully recorded in all but one set of case notes.
- ▶ The history of the presenting complaint was for the most part well documented, although a few factors were occasionally omitted (e.g. precipitating events).
- ▶ Several sets of case notes were poorly set out and the information was difficult to retrieve or understand.

These results highlight some important issues and perhaps evidence of laxity in the recording of psychiatric notes.

Recommendations

- ▶ Pro formas or electronic notes might improve the recording of case notes.
- ▶ Clinicians should be reminded that case notes are legal documents and therefore should always be complete.

Cooper, J. E. & Oates, M. (2003) Assessment: principles of clinical assessment in general psychiatry. In *New Oxford Textbook of Psychiatry* (eds M. G. Gelder, J. J. Lopez-Ibor & N. Andreasen), pp. 62–78. Oxford University Press.

Hampton, J. R., Harrison, M. J., Mitchell, J. R., *et al* (1975) Relative contributions of history-taking, physical examination, and laboratory investigation to diagnosis and management of medical outpatients. *BMJ, ii*, 486–489.

Osborn, G. D., Pike, H., Smith, M., *et al* (2005) Quality of clinical case note entries: how good are we at achieving set standards? *Annals of the Royal College of Surgeons of England*, **87**, 458–460.

49. Documentation of ward reviews

Nuruz Zaman

Setting

This audit is relevant to all psychiatric specialties and can be adapted for out-patient reviews.

Background

Medical note-keeping is an important part of clinical practice. It provides a record of patient progress and continuity of care, a basis for communication within the multidisciplinary team, a record for coding and research, and is a medico-legal requirement. Guidance from the General Medical Council (GMC) (2006) states: 'Keep clear, accurate, legible and contemporaneous patient records which report the relevant clinical findings, the decision made, the information given to the patients and any drugs or other treatment prescribed'. There are no specific guidelines for psychiatric records but in *Good Psychiatric Practice* (2009) the Royal College of Psychiatrists recommends that the GMC guidance is followed.

The Audit Commission's 'payment by results' (PbR) data assurance framework in 2008 found significant levels of error with medical coding. The most common factor contributing to errors was the quality of the source documentation from which the coding data were extracted. This included illegible or poorly structured case notes.

Standards

Following review of published standards and wide consultation, the Health Informatics Unit of the Royal College of Physicians (2009) produced generic medical record-keeping standards. Standard 6 requires that every entry in the medical record is dated, timed (in 24-hour format), legible and signed by the person making the entry. The name and designation of the person making the entry should be legibly printed against the signature. Deletions and alterations should be countersigned, dated and timed.

Method

Data collection

Ten sets of patient notes in each in-patient unit were selected. The entries made on a specified date (a week or two earlier) were examined. Each medical entry should have been legible and was examined for the presence of:

▶ date and time
▶ a record of participants at the review
▶ signature, printed name and designation of the doctor making the entry
▶ where a particular plan had been documented, a further entry to establish that this was carried out (e.g. blood results where blood tests were planned).

Data analysis

The percentage of entries meeting the following standards was calculated:

- presence of a date and time
- list of participants at review
- presence of a signature, printed name and designation of doctor
- legibility of entries
- documentation of the completion of plans.

Resources required

People
This audit can be undertaken by a single doctor.

Time
For 10 sets of notes, around 2 hours should be allowed for data collection.

Results
Completion of the following was good:
- date (97%)
- signature (97%)
- printed name (87%).

Performance in other parameters was less good:
- legibility (73%)
- plan completion (70%)
- list of participants at review (66%)
- designation of doctor (40%)
- time of entry (23%).

The high rate of documenting the date, signature and name was encouraging. With such basic data being audited, the expectation would, though, be for better performance overall. There was a clear requirement for improved documentation of the time of review, participants involved in review, designation of the note-taker and documentation of the completion of plans.

Recommendations
- Promoting improved awareness and training on the importance of medical note-keeping. In particular noting the need for documentation of the missing information and recognition of the importance of legibility.
- Auditing of documentation should be carried out on a regular basis, to monitor quality, especially with the regular change-over of junior doctors.
- Consider further audits into the quality of the content of notes.

Audit Commission (2008) *PbR Data Assurance Framework 2007/08: Findings from the First Year of the National Clinical Coding Audit Programme*. Audit Commission.

General Medical Council (2006) *Good Medical Practice*. GMC. Available at http://www.gmc-uk.org/guidance/good_medical_practice.asp (accessed October 2010).

Royal College of Physicians (2009) *Improving Clinical Records and Clinical Coding Together. A Project with the Audit Commission*. Available at http://www.rcplondon.ac.uk/clinical-standards/hiu/Documents/200908-Improving-clinical-records-and-clinical-coding-together-v1.0.pdf (accessed October 2010).

Royal College of Psychiatrists (2009) *Good Psychiatric Practice*. Royal College of Psychiatrists. Available at http://www.rcpsych.ac.uk/files/pdfversion/CR154.pdf (accessed October 2010).

50. Letters to general practitioners

Tanja-Sabine Schumm and Linda Findlay

Setting

This audit was within intellectual disability psychiatry but may be relevant to out-patient follow-up clinics in other areas in psychiatry.

Background

Out-patient letters between secondary and primary care are an important form of communication. With restructuring of mental health services and closure of large psychiatric hospitals, an increasing number of patients with intellectual disability and mental health problems have been resettled in the community and are under the care of general practitioners (GPs). This audit examined the quality of letters that were sent out to GPs after their patients were assessed in follow-up clinics.

Standards

A literature review was performed (sources are listed below) and, following discussion with colleagues, standards were defined. The following were to be included in all letters:

▶ patient's demographics
▶ date of clinic
▶ patient's diagnosis
▶ update on symptoms/problems
▶ current mental state
▶ current medication and dosage
▶ opinion/summary
▶ follow-up arrangements.

Other points which could be considered are:

▶ copies sent to multidisciplinary team or patient
▶ letters are sent within a certain time after the appointment
▶ comment on quality of life.

Method

Data collection

Out-patient letters to GPs were examined against the defined standards. Medical secretaries had a list of all patients who attended out-patient clinics for follow-up and were able to provide the letters. Alternatively, out-patient follow-up letters were found in patients' clinical notes.

Data analysis

The percentage of patients for whom the standards were met was calculated.

Resources required

People

One person can undertake this audit.

Time

The duration of data collection will depend on the time required to access the letters and the length of the out-patient letters. Data collection from 50 letters (at an average length of half an A4 page) took about 2 hours.

Results

The documentation of demographics, date of clinic, update on symptoms/ problems and follow-up arrangements was very good. Within the letters collected, 71% reported the patient's medication, including dosage, 57% their mental state, 16% a diagnosis and 27% an opinion/summary.

After implementing the steps below, documentation had improved dramatically at the time of a re-audit.

Recommendations

▶ All medical staff in the department should be informed of the audit results and consulted regarding the introduction of a template letter.

▶ A template letter with the following subheadings should be introduced:

 ▷ patient details and date of clinic appointment

 ▷ diagnosis (ICD–10)

 ▷ known comorbid medical disorders

 ▷ update on symptoms/problems

 ▷ mental state examination

 ▷ opinion/summary

 ▷ recommendations

 ▷ medication (full list of current medications and reasons for any change in medication)

 ▷ other

 ▷ follow-up arrangements.

Davey, C., Desai, A. B. & Shajahan, P. M. (2006) Are we giving general practitioners what they want from psychiatric out-patient review letters? *Scottish Medical Journal*, **51**(4), 49.

Markar, T. N. (2002) Communication between psychiatrists and general practitioners in learning disability – a clinical audit. *British Journal of Developmental Disabilities*, **48**, 107–112.

Pullen, I. M. & Yellowlees, A. J. (1985) Is communication improving between general practitioners and psychiatrists? *BMJ*, **290**, 31–33.

Thalayasingam, S., Alexander, R. T. & Singh, I. (1999) Audit on letters from psychiatrists to general practitioners following assessment of patients with learning disabilities in follow-up clinics. *British Journal of Developmental Disabilities*, **45**, 123–127.

51. Medication alerts in electronic patient records

Zeid Mohammed and Iain McKinnon

Setting

This audit is relevant to all psychiatric specialties and can be modified where electronic records are not in use.

Background

In August 2008, a new electronic patient record system, PARIS, was introduced to the Tees, Esk and Wear Valleys NHS Foundation Trust. It was intended to replace hard-copy case notes, providing all clinical information in an easily accessible form to clinical teams. Some of this information relates to 'clinical alerts', which warn clinicians about significant risks associated with the patient. The decision to add a clinical alert must be based on a specific incident or on expression of a clearly identifiable concern, and the risk needs to be made explicit to other practitioners as soon as they access the record.

As many psychiatric patients have physical comorbidities requiring treatment and others are on high doses of psychotropic medications, a specific 'significant medication alert' can be created for a patient where relevant. The audit aimed to ensure that this alert had been applied appropriately according to the trust's electronic records policy.

Standards

According to the trust's policy, a 'significant medication alert' is required when a patient is taking one of the following:

- high dose of antipsychotics
- high dose of antidepressants
- lithium
- warfarin
- insulin
- methotrexate.

A high dose of antipsychotic/antidepressant is any dose above the maximum dose stated in either *The Maudsley Prescribing Guidelines* (Taylor *et al*, 2007) or the *British National Formulary* (Joint Formulary Committee, 2009).

Method

Data collection

All patients within the trust's learning disability department were identified. A random sample of patients was then selected. The patient's current medications were checked by scrutinising out-patient letters and the discharge summary uploaded on the system. The presence or absence of a 'significant medication alert' was recorded on a data collection sheet.

Data analysis

Patient records were analysed against the following criteria:

- adequate documentation of medication
- the presence or absence of a 'significant medication alert'
- if an alert was present, that there was appropriate documentation of the medication
- where an alert was no longer relevant (e.g. after discontinuation of the medication) that the alert had been deactivated
- the absence of an alert where there should have been one.

Resources required

People

It is suggested that this audit is undertaken by at least two people, owing to the amount of information collected.

Time

For a sample of 115 patients, data collection took around 2 days.

Results

- In 16 patients out of 115, it was not possible to tell what non-psychotropic medication was prescribed – information was absent from the discharge summary and out-patient letters.
- Ten patients had a 'significant medication alert' documented.
- Of the ten, nine patients had the type of medication documented and one did not.
- There were no instances of alerts having been left on the system where they were no longer appropriate (i.e. deactivation of alerts was occurring).
- Eleven patients who were on significant medication (ten on lithium, one on insulin) had no medication alert.

Recommendations

- Clinicians should initiate a review of medication alerts.
- A full medication history should be included in the assessment, in the discharge summary and in out-patient letters.
- The minimum information available on all patients should include a note of their most recent medication and a copy of the most recent out-patient letter (if applicable).
- Clozapine should be included in the list of significant medications.
- In trusts with no electronic records, similar mechanisms should be introduced by documentation on prescription cards and liaison with the pharmacy.

Joint Formulary Committee (2009) *British National Formulary* (58th edition). British Medical Association & Royal Pharmaceutical Society of Great Britain.

Taylor, D., Paton, C. & Kerwin, R. (2007) *The Maudsley Prescribing Guidelines* (9th edition). Informa Healthcare.

52. Risk assessment: forms for in-patients

Neil Masson, Ashley Liew, John Taylor and Frank McGuigan

Setting

This audit is relevant for in-patient mental health services where standardised in-patient risk assessment tools are used for all patients admitted to hospital.

Background

The increasing expectation on all mental health professionals to identify, appraise and manage risk has led to the introduction of generic risk assessment forms, which are now used in the majority of trusts in the UK and are often mandatory for all in-patients (Higgins *et al*, 2005).

Standards

The standard used for this audit comes from the Department of Health's *Best Practice in Managing Risk* (2007), which advocates the use of tools in risk assessment and management. The standard should be that all psychiatric in-patients have adequately completed risk assessment forms.

Method

Data collection

The case notes of all current in-patients on a specified day were reviewed. A standardised form was used to collect anonymised data on the following variables:

▶ patient age and gender
▶ date and time of admission and admission ward
▶ detention status
▶ admitting doctor
▶ presence of an adequately completed risk assessment tool.

Data analysis

The main outcome measure was the percentage of in-patients with an adequately completed risk assessment form. This ranged from a fully completed form, to an incomplete form, to no form at all. Data were collected on how well each section of the form was completed so that deficiencies in particular areas could be highlighted. Chi-squared tests were used to determine the relationship between incomplete forms and variables such as patient age, gender, admission ward, date and time of admission, detention status and admitting doctor.

Resources required

People

The number of people involved will depend on the number of wards that are included in the audit. If the risk tool is used across a number of hospitals in a trust, then it would be useful to audit all of these hospitals at the same time, which would need more than one person.

Time

It is estimated that at least 6 hours should be dedicated to reviewing the case notes of 40 in-patients.

Results

The percentage of fully completed risk assessment forms was low. There was no association between rates of completion of forms and whether the form was completed during working hours or out of hours, the detention status of the patient or the gender of the patient. The first intervention below resulted in improved completion rates 2 months later and this improvement was sustained after the second intervention, 6 months after that.

Recommendations

▶ A memorandum should be sent to all clinical staff highlighting the importance of the risk assessment tool and giving a brief synopsis of the results of the audit. The results of the audit should additionally be presented to clinical staff, followed by an interactive discussion on risk assessment.

▶ The risk assessment tool should be included within a standardised admission pack comprising all the forms that need to be completed when a patient is admitted to hospital.

Department of Health (2007) *Best Practice in Managing Risk: Principles and Guidance for Best Practice in the Assessment and Management of Risk to Self and Others in Mental Health Services*. DH. Available at http://www.library.nhs.uk/mentalHealth/ViewResource.aspx?resID=266056 (accessed October 2010).

Higgins, N., Watts, D., Bindman, J., *et al* (2005) Assessing violence risk in general adult psychiatry. *Psychiatric Bulletin*, **29**, 131–133.

53. Risk assessment: medium-secure unit

Ruth Scally

Setting

This audit is particularly relevant in forensic settings but also applies to any adult psychiatric service, both in- and out-patient.

Background

An assessment of the risks posed by patients, whether self-harm, absconding or violence to others, should be recorded in the patient's notes. In the trust audited, these assessments are based on the HCR-20 (Historical Clinical Risk),a 20-item structured clinical risk assessment tool that is widely used in forensic settings (Khiroya *et al*, 2009).

Standards

The National Institute for Health and Clinical Excellence (NICE) has produced a guideline (2005) on the short-term management of disturbed and violent behaviour in in-patient psychiatric settings. It states that 'there should be an effective risk assessment and risk management plan … in the case notes of each service user at high risk and that this should be reviewed on a regular basis'. For the purposes of this audit, this was interpreted as all patients having an HCR-20 form in their notes, which had been reviewed within the past 12 months.

Method

Data collection

The medical records of all in-patients on one specific day were reviewed and the following data collected:

▶ whether an HCR-20 form was present in the notes
▶ whether it had been completed
▶ whether it had been reviewed in the past 12 months
▶ the number of disciplines involved in the risk assessment (i.e. whether it was a multidisciplinary assessment).

In addition the length of stay of each patient was noted.

This audit was conducted in combination with an audit of risk assessment documentation for the care programme approach (CPA) within the trust.

Data analysis

The percentage of sets of case notes meeting the standards was calculated for:

▶ those with an HCR-20 form
▶ those that were complete
▶ those that had been reviewed in the preceding 12 months.

The number (and nature) of disciplines involved was counted and displayed in a bar chart.

Resources required

People

Depending on the size of the population being studied, this audit would be suitable for one or two people, of any discipline.

Time

About 4 hours should be allowed for an audit of 90 patients.

Results

Approximately two-thirds of patients had an HCR-20 form present in their case notes, but only just over half had a fully completed document. Invariably it was the formulation that had been omitted. The majority of assessments were completed by more than one person and the full range of professions was represented.

Recommendations

- ▶ Risk assessments should be reviewed as part of the 6-monthly CPA review.
- ▶ The audit should be repeated after 12 months.

Khiroya, K., Weaver, T. & Maden, T. (2009) Use and perceived utility of structured violence risk assessments in English medium secure forensic units. *Psychiatric Bulletin*, **33**, 129–132.

National Institute for Health and Clinical Excellence (2005) *Violence: The Short-Term Management of Disturbed/Violent Behaviour in In-patient Settings and Emergency Departments* (CG25). NICE. Available at http://guidance.nice.org.uk/CG25 (accessed October 2010).

V. Service provision

Early intervention teams
Emergency department: attendance
Information for in-patients on their rights
Interpreters
Liaison psychiatry: response time to referrals
Multi-agency working
Personal searches
Prison equivalence
Prison-to-hospital transfers
Seven-day follow-up
Substance misuse: the Treatment Outcomes Profile
Transition from 'choice' to 'partnership' in the Choice
    and Partnership Approach
Transition planning in attention-deficit hyperactivity disorder
Violent incidents: management
Waiting times

54. Early intervention teams

Vanessa Pinfold, Jo Smith and David Shiers

Setting

This audit will be relevant to all psychiatrists, though those working in and with services for early intervention in psychosis (EI) will find it especially useful.

Background

EI is a key component of modern mental health services in England (Department of Health, 2000). It involves the specialist support of people with first-episode psychosis aged 14–35 years and their families and comprises three concepts: the early detection of psychosis; a reduction in the duration of untreated psychosis; the importance of the first 3–5 years following onset (the critical period) for later biological, psychological and social outcomes.

Standards

The *Mental Health Policy Implementation Guide* (PIG) (Department of Health, 2001) provides a model for EI. On the basis of this model, the Department of Health specified eight minimum fidelity criteria against which providers could self-assess local EI services. These were expanded to give ten standards against which services were assessed in this audit:

- stand-alone service model
- dedicated consultant psychiatrist input
- full age range (14–35 years)
- care provided for up to 3 years
- assertive community outreach work
- extended opening hours
- case-loads of 10–15 per care coordinator
- adolescent provision
- primary care referral
- designated access to acute beds.

These criteria are included in the Department of Health's autumn assessment local delivery plan (LDP) returns (see also Tiffin & Glover, 2007).

Method

Data collection

Service managers within EI teams should ensure there is a system in place to document minimum data on all patients under their care and that operational descriptors accurately describe the service model. Information on patient age, referral source and interventions received were obtained from patient case files. Service managers should therefore be able to provide the data required within the audit 'window'. A bespoke tool was used in the present audit, but an EI audit pro forma is available online as part of the LDP autumn assessment to assist efficiency of data collection and analysis (http://www.ic.nhs.uk/services/mental-health/mental-health-minimum-dataset-mhmds).

Data analysis

▶ Individual service returns were collated to give a national overview of the current state of EI service development in England. Data were also available for each of the eight health regions in England. The data can be collated on a more local level for individual services.

▶ A simple numeric fidelity rating based on number of criteria met (yes = 1; no = 0) was used to assess mean minimum fidelity based on the ten criteria expanded from the EI PIG and outlined in the standards above.

Resources required

People

The audit can be carried out by one central coordinator but requires assistance from regional EI leads and service managers. Locally it could be conducted by one person.

Time

If the data required are routinely recorded and accessible to the service manager, the audit would take 30 minutes to complete.

Results

In 2005 there were 117 EI teams across England. Of these, 75% described themselves as adherent to the policy implementation guide, but the degree of fidelity was variable. The mean fidelity score was 6.44 (median 6; range 1–10). The audit revealed national coverage of EI, but with one-third of the population without a local EI service in 2005. Access to acute in-patient beds was variable, as were extended opening hours in the service.

Recommendations

▶ The audit gives a guide to EI services concerning key areas for development to improve model fidelity, to aid service planning and improvement programmes.

▶ The audit results were fed back to the Department of Health to assess progress in relation to EI policy implementation and fidelity to the EI PIG. The data informed the subsequent EI recovery plan (Department of Health, 2006).

▶ Information relating to adolescent bed provision was used to inform actions in relation to the provision of age-appropriate in-patient care.

▶ Recommendations for staff training were made (Pinfold *et al*, 2007).

Department of Health (2000) *The NHS Plan: A Plan for Investment, A Plan for Reform*. The Stationery Office. Available at http://www.dh.gov.uk/en/Publicationsandstatistics/Publications/PublicationsPolicyAndGuidance/DH_4002960 (accessed October 2010).

Department of Health (2001) *Mental Health Policy Implementation Guide*. DH.

Department of Health (2006) *Early Intervention Recovery Plan*. DH.

Pinfold, V., Smith, J. & Shiers, D. (2007) Audit of early intervention in psychosis service development in England in 2005. *Psychiatric Bulletin*, 31, 7–10.

Tiffin, P. & Glover, G. (2007) From commitment to reality: early intervention in psychosis services in England. *Early Intervention in Psychiatry*, 1, 104–107.

55. Emergency department: attendance

Jim Bolton

Setting

This audit may be particularly relevant to liaison psychiatry services and other mental health services that accept referrals from emergency departments.

Background

The NHS Plan introduced an aim to reduce waiting times for patients attending emergency departments (Department of Health, 2000). This audit aimed to measure the proportion of patients referred to mental health services who remained in an emergency department for longer than 4 hours and to identify the reasons for prolonged attendance.

Standards

The standard was derived from the NHS Plan, which stipulated that, from 2004 onwards, over 98% of patients attending an emergency department should have completed their attendance episode within 4 hours (Department of Health, 2000). This time includes any assessment and management by specialist services that occurs in the emergency department. The standard set was that over 98% of referrals to liaison psychiatry should have an attendance time of under 4 hours.

Method

Data collection

Emergency department records were collected for all patients who were referred by the emergency department to the liaison psychiatry service over a 3-month period. For each attendance, the total attendance time was calculated. Where the attendance time was over 4 hours, the records were examined to identify the main reasons for a prolonged attendance.

Data analysis

Two time intervals were calculated, between:
- booking into the emergency department and assessment by a doctor
- referral to the liaison psychiatry service and psychiatric assessment.

For both intervals, an arbitrary duration of greater than 1 hour was recorded as contributing to a prolonged attendance.

Resources required

People

Cooperation is required from emergency department staff in order to collect patient records. It is suggested that the audit is undertaken by at least two people, owing to the amount information to be collected and the possible need to confer when points are uncertain. It is recommended that the auditors are clinical staff who are familiar with clinical records and emergency department care.

Time

The audit should be conducted over a long enough period to gain a representative number of cases (e.g. 3 months). It is estimated that data collection would take 15–20 hours.

Results

During the 3 months of the audit, 32 patients were referred to liaison psychiatry from the emergency department. In 14 instances (44%) the attendance time was longer than 4 hours. The main reasons identified for prolonged attendance in the emergency department were:

▶ over 1 hour between attendance at the emergency department and assessment by a doctor

▶ over 1 hour between referral to and assessment by the liaison psychiatry service

▶ patients awaiting the results of blood investigations following an overdose

▶ patients requiring psychiatric admission awaiting transport

▶ patient intoxication with alcohol

▶ patient requiring medical observation following an overdose.

The findings of the audit led to a number of service improvements in both the emergency department and the liaison psychiatry service. Subsequent audit cycles demonstrated a significant improvement in attendance times.

Recommendations

▶ Emergency department referrals should be prioritised by liaison psychiatry, with assessment within 1 hour of referral.

▶ An observation ward should be established next to the emergency department, such that patients requiring prolonged attendance for medical reasons can be temporarily admitted to the general hospital.

▶ Guidelines and protocols should facilitate assessment of patients with mental health problems attending the emergency department, in order to increase staff confidence and to minimise assessment times.

Department of Health (2000) *The NHS Plan*. DH (www.dh.gov.uk/en/Publicationsandstatistics/Publications/PublicationsPolicyAndGuidance/DH_4010198).

56. Information for in-patients on their rights

Alice Lomax and Frances Raphael

Setting

This audit is most suited to general adult psychiatry but would also be relevant to other in-patient services.

Background

The experience of being an in-patient is intended to be supportive, containing and fundamentally therapeutic. However, aspects of being a psychiatric in-patient are highly stressful, such as the inability to come and go without restriction. Article 5(1) of the European Convention on Human Rights states that everyone has the right to liberty, but in the case of people who are mentally ill detention may be lawful. Psychiatric staff face difficulties balancing the right to freedom with safety and their duty of care. The practice of locking 'open wards' has increased recently, in an apparent reversal of the ethos of psychiatric care over the past three decades, when psychiatry began to move towards unlocked wards and community care (*Lancet*, 1976).

Section 132 of the Mental Health Act (MHA) details hospital managers' duty to inform patients detained under the Act of their rights. There is no legal duty to inform voluntary patients but it would be good practice. Rogers *et al* (1993) found that most informal in-patients felt that they had not received enough information about their treatment. Sugarman & Moss (1994) found that only half of informal patients thought they were legally allowed to leave hospital and only 47% thought they could legally refuse treatment.

Standards

These were based on the European Convention on Human Rights and the Mental Health Act. All patients should:
▶ know their status
▶ be offered a ward welcome pack.
All detained patients should:
▶ know under which section they are detained
▶ be offered a leaflet and explanation from staff about their rights.
All voluntary patients should:
▶ have had their rights explained or been offered a leaflet
▶ know they have the right to refuse treatment.
No voluntary patients should be kept on a ward against their will without an MHA assessment.

Method

Data collection

All available patients on in-patient wards who verbally consented were interviewed. Those lacking capacity to consent to interview were excluded.

Data analysis

Cases meeting the above standards were expressed as a percentage of the total.

Resources

People

This audit can be performed by a single person.

Time

For three in-patient wards, 1 week should be allowed.

Results

- ► Of the voluntary patients, 4% thought that they were detained (1 patient), 42% did not know and 54% knew they were not detained.
- ► Twelve detained patients (86%) knew their status, while two (14%) did not. Eleven knew which section they were detained under.
- ► Eight (21%) of all patients interviewed had received a ward welcome pack but only five had read it.
- ► Half of the detained patients said they had not been informed of their rights.
- ► Nine (64%) said they had been given a leaflet, of whom four had read it, and five (36%) said none had been offered.
- ► Three voluntary patients (13%) said they had had their rights explained to them, and only one had received a leaflet (and read it).
- ► Nine (38%) thought they would not be allowed to go home, while six (25%) did not know.
- ► Eight (33%) thought they would not be allowed a short period off the ward (e.g. to go to the shops or a café), while three (13%) did not know.
- ► Fifteen voluntary patients (63%) had not asked staff if they could leave.
- ► Nine voluntary patients (38%) knew they could legally refuse a treatment; nine (38%) did not know and six (25%) thought they could not refuse.
- ► No one interviewed described being physically stopped from leaving the ward without an MHA assessment.
- ► No one believed they could not leave simply because the door was locked.

Recommendations

- ► A survey of staff would clarify their understanding of patient rights and then training could be provided as needed.
- ► An information leaflet could be developed and be given to all voluntary in-patients.
- ► Further work should be done on improving information giving with staff and patient groups.
- ► The audit cycle should be completed by a re-audit within 18 months.

Lancet (1976) Who's for the locked ward? [Editorial] *Lancet, i,* 461.

Rogers, A., Pilgrim, D. & Lacey, R. (1993) *Experiencing Psychiatry: Users' Views of Services.* Macmillan.

Sugarman, P. & Moss, J. (1994) The rights of voluntary patients in hospital. *Psychiatric Bulletin,* 18, 269–271.

57. Interpreters

Barnett Musiime

Setting

This audit is relevant in all subspecialties and in all psychiatric settings.

Background

Communicating with patients who do not speak English as a first language is a common challenge and yet it is impossible to provide high-quality mental health services without excellent communication between mental health staff and patients. It is worth noting that the Royal College of Psychiatrists does not currently have guidelines on working through interpreters.

Standards

Standards were obtained from the Victorian Transcultural Psychiatry Unit (VTPU). These are generally acceptable standards which were published in 2006 in Australia. They give guidance on booking interpreters and the use of interpreters before and during the interview, and requesting feedback after the interview:

▶ Appointments should be for 1.5 hours and time should be used to maximum effect.
▶ The patient and the interpreter should be matched as closely as possible regarding language and dialect, education, ethnic origin, religion and gender preferences.
▶ During the consultation, chairs should be arranged such that the interpreter is next to the health worker, opposite patient (this may have to be adapted according to the size of the group).
▶ The health worker should keep control of the meeting and speak directly to the patient.
▶ The health worker should use short sentences and expect everything said in the room to be interpreted.
▶ A 'code word' can be used to stop the meeting if the patient wishes to.
▶ The worker should give the interpreter feedback after the meeting and ask for feedback in return.

The target is that these standards are met for all patients seen through interpreters.

Method

Data collection

A list of trust employees was obtained from human resources. A question-naire, developed to reflect the above standards (and that included demographic information), was distributed to staff (this could include any staff group with patient contact or only doctors) either in person or through the internal mail system.

Data analysis

The percentage of staff who reported meeting the above standards was calculated.

Resources required

People

This audit should be undertaken by two people, owing to the amount of information that needs to be collected and analysed.

Time

It is estimated that for 50 completed questionnaires it would take around 8 weeks to collect and 3 hours to analyse all the data.

Results

- Out of the 50 questionnaires sent out, 30 (60%) were returned. Thirteen members of staff (43%) had seen at least five patients with an interpreter in the preceding 3 months and six (20%) had seen over 15 patients during the same period with an interpreter.
- Twenty-three respondents (77%) were able to keep control of the meeting most of the time.
- Thirteen (43%) were able to speak directly to the patient most of the time.
- About a third of clinicians allowed enough time to meet and brief the interpreter before the meeting.
- Seventeen (57%) reassured the patient of confidentiality on every occasion an interpreter was used.
- Ten doctors (33%) were able to ask the interpreter for comments and concerns about the patient's condition on most occasions.
- About a third of clinicians asked for feedback from the interpreter after the meeting and only four (13%) never did so.
- The majority (80%) felt that working through interpreters should be made a part of core psychiatric training.

Recommendations

- Training on the use of interpreters should be included at trainee and senior clinician level, for all staff groups.
- The trust should develop guidelines for working with interpreters, with the assistance of the Diversity organisation.

Victorian Transcultural Psychiatry Unit (2006) *Guidelines for Working Effectively with Interpreters in Mental Health Settings*. VTPU. Available at http://www.vtpu.org.au/docs/interpreter/VTPU_GuidelinesBooklet.pdf (accessed October 2010).

Acknowledgements

Dr Saeed Farooq (locum consultant, Birmingham and Solihull Mental Health Foundation Trust) and Sue Ellis (Clinical Audit Coordinater, Birmingham and Solihull Mental Health Foundation Trust) helped with the original audit.

58. Liaison psychiatry: response time to referrals

Jim Bolton and Nicolette Kaneza

Setting

This audit will be particularly relevant to liaison psychiatry services and mental health services accepting referrals from general hospitals and emergency departments.

Background

In collaboration with other healthcare organisations, the Royal College of Psychiatrists has established quality standards for liaison psychiatry services as part of the Psychiatric Liaison Accreditation Network (PLAN) (Royal College of Psychiatrists, 2009). Timeliness of response to referrals is one quality indicator. This audit informed the setting of the PLAN response time standards.

Standards

The audit standards were developed following agreement by members of the liaison psychiatry service about what would constitute clinically appropriate response times to referrals. This discussion was informed by the 4-hour attendance time target set for emergency departments by the Department of Health for England (Department of Health, 1999). This led to a focus on factors that might unnecessarily delay the management of patients in an emergency department. One such factor is the response time of specialist services to referrals made by emergency department staff.

Following discussion with referrers, referrals were categorised according to the urgency of response required. The standards set for the audit were the maximum response times agreed for each category:

▶ emergency referrals (including all referrals from the emergency department) to be assessed within 1 hour
▶ urgent referrals to be assessed on the same working day
▶ routine referrals to be assessed within 2 working days.

Method

Data collection

The time of referral and the response time by the liaison psychiatry service were recorded for all referrals over a 3-month period. These data were collected by adaptation of the service's pre-existing referral form. In addition to the response time, data were collected on the source of the referral, the primary reason for the referral and the urgency of the referral.

Data analysis

The percentage of patients achieving the standard, and the mean response time and standard deviation, were calculated for each category.

Resources required

People

This audit requires participation by all service members who accept and assess new referrals, in order to ensure that the necessary data are recorded. The audit itself can be conducted by a single person.

Time

The audit should be conducted over a period that allows a sufficient representative sample of referrals to be obtained (e.g. 3 months). It is estimated that data collection would take 10–15 hours.

Results

- Over the 3-month period of the audit, data were collected for 124 referrals.
- Of all referrals, 82% were from the general hospital wards and 18% were from the emergency department.
- The commonest reason for referral from both the wards and emergency department was self-harm.
- For the three categories of referral the response time standards were achieved in all cases.
- The proportion of referrals in each group and the mean response times were as follows:
  - emergency, 25%, 21 minutes (s.d. = 20)
  - urgent, 30%, 70 minutes (s.d. = 86)
  - routine, 45%, 200 minutes (s.d. = 183).

Recommendations

- Although the standards were met during the audit, this was considered to be a sufficiently important measure of the quality of the service to repeat the audit at a later date, particularly with regard to emergency department referrals.
- The categorisation of response times should inform the setting of quality standards for liaison psychiatry services across the UK (Royal College of Psychiatrists, 2009).

Department of Health (1999) *Reforming Emergency Care*. DH.

Royal College of Psychiatrists (2009) *Quality Standards for Liaison Psychiatry Services*. Royal College of Psychiatrists. Available at http://www.rcpsych.ac.uk/pdf/PLAN%20Standards%20First%20Edition%20Sep2009.pdf (accessed October 2010).

59. Multi-agency working

Floriana Coccia

Setting

This audit was performed in a child and adolescent mental health service (CAMHS), but can be adapted to any service where there is frequent interaction with non-mental health organisations such as social services or education.

Background

Multidisciplinary approaches to complex cases referred to CAMHS are both mandated and necessary, but multidisciplinary working is time-consuming and resource intensive, especially where processes are not functioning optimally. CAMHSs are envisioned as providing a mix of direct and indirect (consultation and liaison) services. The approach requires communication between agencies with different backgrounds, roles and working practices. The aim of this audit was to assess the use and outcome of time allocated for this purpose.

Standards

The standards were derived from principles laid down in the National Service Framework (Department of Health, 2004), *Every Child Matters* (Chief Secretary to the Treasury, 2003) and *Good Medical Practice* (General Medical Council, 2006):

▶ Referral pathways, the organisational process and the aims of the consultation should be clear.
▶ Communication, discussion and decisions should be documented and accessible after the consultation.
▶ Attendance should be documented and named workers should be made responsible for recommended actions.

Method

Data collection

The process used to arrange consultations with non-mental health organisations was identified. Notes from those consultations were located to determine the presence of the following:

▶ the attendees and their designations
▶ the discussion, decision and action plans.

Data analysis

The percentages of cases in which information was clearly documented according to the above standards were calculated.

Resources required

People

This audit can be carried out by a single person of any discipline, although in large services more than one person may be required.

Time

The time required will depend on the size of the sample and the process in place locally. In the first stage of the audit, data collection took around 20 hours for 115 potential cases, from which only 12 relevant cases were found. In the second stage only 4 hours was required for 28 potential cases, from which 14 relevant cases were found, with two auditors in each case.

Results

At the start of the audit process, all referrals from education and social services were offered a consultation in the first instance. This decision was made at multidisciplinary allocation meetings, held weekly. A date was booked on a booking sheet by a named staff member, who was then responsible for organising the meeting. When the consultation meeting took place, documentation was made in the relevant case notes.

During the first phase of the audit attempts were made to trace the information back from the booking form and meeting minutes, and then the notes were located. During the second phase, a new spreadsheet was used to identify all consultations that had occurred, cross-referenced with the allocation meeting minutes.

In the first audit 58% (74) of available consultation slots were booked, but only 12 (20%) consultations took place for which notes could be located. Of these, 67% had the attendees recorded, 83% had discussions documented and 75% had decisions and action plans documented.

After the recommendations below were implemented, 97% (28) of slots were booked and notes were found for half of these. In all 14 cases documentation had improved to 100% in all areas (recording of attendees, documentation of discussions, decisions and action plans).

Recommendations

After the first phase of the audit, results were subject to multidisciplinary discussion, at which recommendations for change were proposed. The following changes were implemented:

- The name of the service was clarified.
- The allocation meeting record form was revised.
- The use of a standard consultation documentation form was instituted.
- Dedicated administrative support for the consultation meetings was arranged and one secretary became responsible for administration. She designed and used a spreadsheet program to manage the use of consultation time.

Chief Secretary to the Treasury (2003) *Every Child Matters*. The Stationery Office.

Department of Health (2004) *National Service Framework for Children, Young People and Maternity Services: Mental Health and Psychological Wellbeing of Children and Young People*. Department of Health. Available from http://www.dh.gov.uk/en/Publicationsandstatistics/Publications/PublicationsPolicyAndGuidance/DH_4089114 (accessed October 2010).

General Medical Council (2006) Working in teams. In *Good Medical Practice*. GMC. Available at http://www.gmc-uk.org/guidance/good_medical_practice.asp (accessed October 2010).

60. Personal searches

Floriana Coccia

Setting

This audit is particularly relevant to forensic in-patient services, psychiatric intensive-care units, general in-patient settings and the emergency departments of general hospitals.

Background

The undertaking of necessary and lawful searches of both patients and visitors as well as ward searches by appropriately trained staff can make a valid contribution to the safety of in-patient settings.

Standards

The National Institute for Health and Clinical Excellence (NICE) (2005) has produced a guideline on the conduct of searches as part of the short-term management of disturbed or violent behaviour in in-patient psychiatric settings and emergency departments. The guideline states that each facility should have an operational search policy in place and this should cover the following:

▶ searching patients, their belongings and the environment in which they are accommodated
▶ searching visitors
▶ 'rub down' or personal searching, together with procedures for authorisation in the absence of consent
▶ the circumstances in which a service user physically resists being searched
▶ the routine and random searching of detained service users.

The standards relating to how searches are carried out are as follows:

▶ Searches should be undertaken by appropriately trained staff of the same gender as the patient.
▶ A comprehensive record of every search should be made, including of what is found on the search.
▶ All aspects of the management of disturbed/violent behaviour should be monitored on a regular basis.

Method

Data collection

Searches should be documented on incident forms (e.g. NHS IR1 forms) and these were cross-referenced with multidisciplinary patient notes. The notes and forms were examined to find entries documenting any of the following for each search in a specified time period:

▶ how many searches were conducted within the time period and, where applicable, the reason for the search (categorised as random or triggered by an event)
▶ who conducted the search, whether they were of the same gender as the patient and whether a witness was present

- what was found on the search
- what management plan was put in place as a result.

Data analysis

The proportion of patients subjected to searches for which the following standards were met were calculated:
- documentation of the dates and reasons for the searches
- documentation of who conducted the search and any witness present
- documentation of what was found
- documentation of resulting management plan.

Resources required

People

This audit may be carried out by an individual, although more than one individual may be required if the institution is large.

Time

The estimated time for data collection is 1 hour per ward to search through incident forms and an additional 20 minutes per incident to collect and record the data.

Results

- There was good compliance with the search being conducted by an individual of the same gender as the patient.
- Overall, documentation was poor and there were no records of witnesses being present.

Recommendations

- The search policy should be available to all staff on wards and staff training should occur during induction of new staff.
- Staff should be trained on how to complete incident forms correctly.
- The individual on duty responsible for personal searches should find an appropriate witness.

National Institute for Health and Clinical Excellence (2005) *Violence: The Short-Term Management of Disturbed/Violent Behaviour in In-patient Settings and Emergency Departments* (CG25). NICE. Available at http://guidance.nice.org.uk/CG25 (accessed October 2010).

61. Prison equivalence

Rebekah Bourne

Setting

This audit was conducted within the prison healthcare service, where prisoners may be receiving either in-patient or out-patient care for mental health problems.

Background

Significant changes in the delivery of healthcare in prisons have led to increased expectations of quality of care. Since April 2006, primary care trusts have been responsible for providing healthcare within prisons and these services are subject to the same clinical governance procedures as in the wider National Health Service, under the principle of 'equivalence of care'.

Standards

Standards were obtained from guidelines for the treatment of depression and schizophrenia produced by the National Institute for Health of Clinical Excellence (NICE) (both 2009). Only some of the standards were selected, for their ease of assessment and importance.

Depression

▶ When initiating treatment there should be a documented assessment of symptoms and a risk assessment.
▶ A selective serotonin reuptake inhibitor (SSRI) should be prescribed as the first-line treatment.
▶ Anyone initiated on treatment should be reviewed in 2 weeks.
▶ For continuing treatment there should be regular review of the need for it.

Schizophrenia

▶ When initiating treatment there should be a documented assessment of symptoms and a risk assessment.
▶ Baseline weight and blood glucose level should be recorded.
▶ An atypical antipsychotic should be prescribed as the first-line treatment.
▶ For continuing prescription there should be regular documentation of symptoms and side-effects.

Method

Data collection

The medication cards for all of the inmates were reviewed and those prescribed antidepressants or antipsychotics identified. The inmate medical records of these patients were then reviewed to select those with a diagnosis of depression or schizophrenia; only these patients were included in the audit. The documentation of their first assessment on entry to prison was examined to determine whether the prescription was a new one (i.e. initiated in prison).

The notes were examined to find entries relating to:

▶ documentation of symptoms and risk
▶ rationale for drug selection
▶ recording of baseline weight and blood glucose level (in schizophrenia)
▶ ongoing review of symptoms and treatment.

Data analysis

The percentages of patients with depression and schizophrenia whose care met the above standards were calculated.

Resources required

People

It is suggested that this audit is undertaken by at least four people, owing to the amount of information collected and the number of notes to be reviewed.

Time

For a prison with approximately 1000 inmates, around 150 medical records will need to be reviewed. This is estimated to take four people 10 hours. It is better done in 1 day, owing to the frequency of moves within the prison system.

Results

The quality of inmate medical records was generally poor, with little recording of symptoms or risk assessment. For the management of depression, an SSRI was not used as the first-line treatment in many cases. There was better documentation of the management of schizophrenia and an atypical was always the first-line prescription. However, there was no recording of baseline weight or blood glucose level.

Recommendations

▶ There should be a system for flagging up prisoners at reception into prison who are on antidepressant or antipsychotic medication.
▶ There should be a clear policy for prescribing antidepressants.
▶ There should be a system of baseline and regular monitoring of physical health for those prescribed antipsychotics.

National Institute for Health and Clinical Excellence (2009) *Schizophrenia: Core Interventions in the Treatment and Management of Schizophrenia in Primary and Secondary Care* (CG82). NICE. Available at http://guidance.nice.org.uk/CG82 (accessed October 2010).

National Institute for Health and Clinical Excellence (2009) *Depression in Adults (Update)* (CG90). NICE. Available at http://guidance.nice.org.uk/CG90 (accessed October 2010).

62. Prison-to-hospital transfers

Andrew Forrester

Setting

This audit is relevant to general adult or forensic psychiatrists working in prison in-reach teams.

Background

Prisoners, as a group, present an excess of severe mental illness. In England and Wales, mental health in-reach teams were introduced to the prison estate to assist with high levels of need. However, prison-to-hospital transfer times have been a particular problem, which this audit sought to clarify.

Standards

No standard times for transferring acutely unwell prisoners to hospital were set until relatively recently. In 2006, the Department of Health produced agreed procedures for the transfer of prisoners to and from hospital under sections 47 and 48 of the Mental Health Act. These guidelines initially set a 7-day target for prisoner transfers, later amended to 14 days. The same 14-day target was affirmed in Lord Bradley's 2009 review of people with mental health problems and intellectual disabilities in the criminal justice system. The government later accepted that transfer delays should be reduced to a minimum, but did not confirm the application of the 14-day target. Section 47 of the Mental Health Act allows mentally disordered sentenced prisoners to be transferred to hospital from prison for treatment, while section 48 of the same Act allows the urgent transfer of mentally disordered remand prisoners. The transfer is ordered by the Secretary of State for Justice, if satisfied of the following:

▶ two doctors have provided written evidence (via a pro forma)
▶ the prisoner has a mental disorder (meaning any disorder or disability of the mind)
▶ the mental disorder is of a nature or degree that makes it appropriate for the individual to be detained in a hospital for medical treatment
▶ appropriate medical treatment is available.

Method

Data collection

The audit was designed for use by one or more prison in-reach teams. Before starting, the relevant prison was identified, along with the time period under examination. The following information was collected from prison medical records:

▶ referral date
▶ assessment date
▶ acceptance date
▶ transfer date
▶ level of security of the accepting unit
▶ section of the Mental Health Act used.

Data analysis

Data were entered into a simple referral database, created in spreadsheet software. The spreadsheet was then used to generate basic descriptive statistics.

Resources required

People

This audit can be done by one person.

Time

Approximately 2 hours should be allowed for each week under examination.

Results

Mentally disordered prisoners in London wait 90–100 days for a hospital bed, which is much longer than the 14-day target.

Recommendations

▶ A series of measures should be piloted within the London prison estate to establish whether a significant reduction in prisoner waiting times can be achieved. These could include new posts to work across care pathways, innovative local arrangements, faster remittal to prison and early involvement of commissioners.

▶ It will be important to re-audit to ascertain the relative merits of these pilots.

Bradley, K. (2009) *The Bradley Report (Lord Bradley's Review of People with Mental Health Problems or Learning Disabilities in the Criminal Justice System)*. Department of Health. Available at http://www.dh.gov.uk/prod_consum_dh/groups/dh_digitalassets/documents/digitalasset/dh_098698.pdf (accessed October 2010).

Department of Health (2006) *Invitation to Pilot a National Waiting Time Standard for the Transfer of Acutely Mentally Ill Prisoners*. DH. Available at http://www.dh.gov.uk/en/Publicationsandstatistics/Lettersandcirculars/Dearcolleagueletters/DH_4137261 (accessed October 2010).

63. Seven-day follow-up

Sobia Khan

Setting

This audit would be relevant to in-patient facilities in all specialties of psychiatry.

Background

A patient's move from an in-patient facility to the community has been identified as the period of maximum suicide risk (National Confidential Inquiry into Suicides and Homicides, 2006). A report by the National Confidential Inquiry into Suicides and Homicides suggested several measures to manage this transition safely. One of these is to offer early follow-up. This is also a key performance indicator and national priority for mental health trusts (Department of Health, 2008).

Standards

Standards were obtained from National Confidential Inquiry into Suicides and Homicides (2006) and local trust '7-day follow-up monitoring rules'. The definition of 7-day follow-up is the number of people within adult mental health services under the care programme approach receiving follow-up (by phone or face-to-face) within seven days of discharge from hospital.

The standards applying to the follow-up are:

▶ face-to-face contact with the patient
▶ telephone contact with the patient where explicitly recorded as acceptable
▶ verbal contact with a carer where explicitly recorded as acceptable
▶ verbal contact with another care professional where responsibility for follow-up has been explicitly passed on to another mental healthcare organisation.

For internal monitoring purposes, the 7-day follow-up period is counted from:

▶ the start of any leave period from hospital
▶ the discharge date from hospital where there is no immediately preceding leave period.

For monitoring purposes, leave periods resulting in return to hospital within 7 days were excluded. Contacts on the same day as discharge were counted as 7-day follow-up provided they began after the recorded discharge or leave start time and took place in a domiciliary location. For mental health trusts to retain their 'green status' on this performance indicator, all patients should have received follow-up within 7 days of discharge from hospital.

Method

Data collection

This audit can be performed retrospectively or prospectively. A list of all discharges from the hospital over a specified time was obtained from the medical records department. For a prospective design, an arrangement could be made with medical records to notify the auditor of discharges from hospital on a daily basis. The medical notes of patients were examined to determine:

- whether under care programme approach (CPA)
- date of discharge from the hospital (possibly from the discharge notification)
- date of first contact after discharge.
- nature of contact (face to face, telephone, etc.)
- person contacted (patient, carer, another care professional)
- which professionals were involved in the first contact.

Data analysis

The number of cases meeting the standard were expressed as a proportion of the total.

Resources required

People

This audit can be undertaken by one auditor if the sample size is small. For auditing large numbers two people may be involved.

Time

For a sample size of 50, data collection can take up to 2 days.

Results

The percentage of patients who received post-discharge follow-up within 7 days was 90%. The majority of contact occurred with the patient and was face to face. After implementation of the recommendations below, the percentage increased to 100% in a prospective re-audit 12 months later.

Recommendations

- The results of this audit should be circulated among all community staff.
- Clinical teams should be reminded of the importance of the 7-day standard.
- The arrangements for the first follow-up should be documented on the discharge notification sheet for ease of monitoring.

Department of Health (2008) Guidance on the Standard NHS Contract for Mental Health and Learning Disability Services. DH (www.dh.gov.uk/en/Publicationsandstatistics/Publications/PublicationsPolicyAndGuidance/DH_091451).

National Confidential Inquiry into Suicides and Homicides (2006) *Avoidable Deaths: Five Year Report of the National Confidential Inquiry into Suicide and Homicide by People with Mental Illness*. University of Manchester.

64. Substance misuse: Treatment Outcomes Profile

Jason Luty

Setting

This audit is relevant to psychiatrists working in substance misuse services.

Background

The Treatment Outcomes Profile (TOP) was developed by the National Treatment Agency for Substance Misuse at the Department of Health and introduced in 2007. It is a single-page questionnaire completed by clinicians following an interview with patients attending substance misuse services. It attempts to measure the amount of illicit drugs used by patients as well as patients' criminal activity and physical and mental health. It must be completed every 3 months for all patients in drug treatment services in England. The results are used to assess the effectiveness of these services.

Standards

Standards for TOP form completion are available from the National Treatment Agency for Substance Misuse:

▶ The TOP should be completed within 2 weeks either side of the date when a patient started structured drug treatment.

▶ It is good practice to conduct regular care plan reviews; these are usually completed in 12 week (3-month) cycles. It is recommended that the TOP is completed as part of this process.

▶ The TOP should be completed within 2 weeks either side of the date when the patient exits structured treatment.

The national standard is 100% for this and funding is dependent on submitting this information to the commissioners (the local drug action teams). In this audit a threshold for TOP compliance of 80% was considered an appropriate standard to reach. This means that a TOP was expected at each treatment stage for at least 80% of the patients who were accessing, retained in or exiting structured drug treatment.

Method

Data collection

Records for all patients in the community substance misuse services within the trust were audited, to ensure the TOP form was properly completed. Information was collected from the patients' medical records, which contained the completed TOP forms.

Data analysis

The primary outcome was the proportion of patients who had a properly completed TOP form.

Resources required

People

Three people are likely to be needed in a service with 200 patients. The audit does not require multidisciplinary involvement, but this can be considered.

Time

The audit can be completed within 1 week if auditors can commit to it full time. In larger services or with part-time commitment, a few weeks should be allowed for completion of the audit.

Results

▶ TOP forms were inspected for 200 patients, of which 86% were fully completed. This was the primary finding. The completion rate was as good as can reasonably be expected and it was not thought necessary to complete the audit cycle in an attempt to increase the completion rate.

▶ The secondary outcomes showed that some of the information on the TOP form had to be invalid, particularly with respect to reporting criminal behaviour. For example, 67% of subjects had no declared funding for illicit drug use in the previous month (despite spending a mean of £988), but also had denied having any paid employment and had denied any criminal activity.

▶ The audit revealed that the section on crime in the TOP form is unreliable and invalid and the forms should therefore be withdrawn.

Recommendations

The trust did not implement any changes as a result of the audit as the completion rates were already high. Unfortunately, the TOP form has been produced by the National Treatment Agency for Substance Misuse. Despite the defects in the TOP form that were revealed by the audit, only the Department of Health is capable of modifying or changing the form. This was recommended in the article that was subsequently published in *Psychiatric Bulletin* (Easow *et al*, 2009).

Easow, J., Varughese, S. & Luty, J. (2009) Criminally invalid: the Treatment Outcome Profile (TOP) form for substance misuse. *Psychiatric Bulletin*, 33, 404–406.

National Treatment Agency for Substance Misuse. Treatment Outcomes Profile (TOP). Available at http://www.nta.nhs.uk/who-healthcare-top.aspx (accessed October 2010).

65. Transition to 'partnership' in the Choice and Partnership Approach

Caroline Fell

Setting

This audit is useful to those who work in a child and adolescent mental health service (CAMHS) where the Choice and Partnership Approach (CAPA) is used.

Background

The CAPA is a clinical system that is widely used in CAMHS throughout the UK, Australia and New Zealand. It is a system that helps the team do the right thing with the right people and at the right time (York & Kingsbury, 2009).

There are three main components in CAPA and they are choice, partnership, and core and specialist work. The last is the 'bread and butter' and the more specialist and therapeutic work in CAMHS, but the concept of choice and partnership is unique to CAPA.

- *Choice.* Children and families make informed choices about what services and interventions may be useful to them. There is a focus on engagement and clinicians need to help the families and young person reach a 'choice point' at the end of the initial appointment (when a partnership appointment is booked with a clinician with the best skills to help).
- *Partnership.* Partnership work represents the bulk of the intervention and can be done by most CAMHS clinicians with generic skills, together with extended skills that can give the partnership appointments a specific 'flavour'. All 'partnership' clinicians need five core treatment skills (assessment, behavioural, cognitive, dynamic and systemic) and 'choice' clinicians need to consider the spread of these skills when offering the family or young person a partnership appointment.
- The change of clinician from 'choice' to 'partnership' is an integral part of the CAPA process and an important theme.

Standards

The recommendations by the founders of CAPA (York & Kingsbury, 2009) regarding the choice appointment for the family or young person who is progressing to partnership are as follows:

- Children and families make an informed choice about what services and interventions will be useful to them, giving them autonomy.
- The focus is on engagement with change, not the clinician.
- Clinicians should facilitate this using their 'expertise'.
- A 'choice point' is reached at end of the choice appointment.
- The choice clinician is changed for the partnership clinician.

Method

Data collection

A questionnaire was created and given to all choice clinicians. The questionnaire was completed if the young person or family were progressing to partnership.

It was audited over a 3-month period. The questionnaire asked the following questions:

- Has the work or intervention that you feel necessary for this young person/ family been discussed with them at the choice appointment?
- Was the young person/family asked what skills or 'personality traits' they would like in their partnership clinician?
- Does your young person/family know of the change in clinician for their partnership appointment at the end of today's meeting?
- Why did you choose the specific clinician that you have assigned for partnership work?
- Are you aware of the core work and specialist work that this specific clinician can offer? Please specify core skills and specialist skills.
- How quickly will your young person/family be seen in partnership?
- Is there anything that you wish was different to ease the transfer of the young person/family from choice to partnership?

Data analysis

The feedback from the questions was analysed and reflected upon for each specific team.

Resources required

People

Usually only one person is required to review the questionnaires.

Time

Analysing data takes approximately 10 minutes per questionnaire audited.

Results

In general, the 'ethos' of CAPA was maintained, and results were positive regarding facilitation of informed choice to the family/young person. When stating the specialist skills of clinicians, they all seemed appropriate, and the majority of cases were seen within 4 weeks. Although time is not stated in the guidelines, it was in keeping with trust policy. The main weakness in the team's process of going from choice to partnership was the understanding of the clinician's skills.

Recommendations

- All partnership appointments should be entered in the diary in advance, giving choice clinicians a full understanding of the team's availability.
- A 'skill profile' of all partnership clinicians should be created. This would help educate the team on colleagues' skills and expertise in the five domains, and improve discussion in choice appointments with the family/ young person.
- The team as a whole should be educated in the themes and structure of CAPA.

York, A. & Kingsbury, S. (2009) The Choice and Partnership Approach: A Guide to CAPA. CAMHS Network. See also http://www.camhsnetwork.co.uk/index.htm (accessed 2010).

66. Transition planning in attention-deficit hyperactivity disorder

Katherine Telford

Setting

This audit can take place in child and adolescent psychiatry for patients diagnosed with attention-deficit hyperactivity disorder (ADHD) where the guideline from the National Institute for Health and Clinical Excellence (NICE) (2008) recommends transition planning.

Background

Over recent years, ADHD has been re-conceptualised as a chronic disorder (Willoughby, 2003; Faraone *et al*, 2006). Using DSM–IV criteria for the definition of ADHD, the rate of persistence is about 15% at age 25. Using an alternative definition of impairing symptoms of ADHD that do not meet the full criteria of ADHD (partial remission) the persistence rate is 40–60% (National Institute for Health and Clinical Excellence, 2008). Young people who have had their ADHD managed by a child and adolescent mental health service (CAMHS) are likely to require ongoing treatment for ADHD from adult mental health services. This transition of care requires planning.

Standards

The following points of the NICE guideline on ADHD were audited:
▶ Patients with ADHD should be reassessed at school-leaving age to establish the need for continuing treatment.
▶ During the transition to adult services, a formal meeting involving CAMHS and/or paediatrics and adult psychiatric services should be considered.
▶ The young person and, when appropriate, the parent or carer should be involved in the planning and full information should be provided to the young person about adult services.

Method

Data collection

All patients of school-leaving age (i.e. in year 11 or more at UK secondary school) who had ADHD were identified. This stage was reliant on the department having some system of recording patients by diagnosis. The audit can either look only at cases still open, or can also include patients who are in the same age cohort and who have ADHD but have been discharged. This makes the audit more useful in terms of identifying unmet needs. Notes were reviewed to find evidence of transition planning documented either in letters or minutes of meetings or in written records to establish the following:
▶ the transition to adult services or the need for ongoing management from age 18 had been discussed with the parent(s)
▶ the transition to adult services or the need for ongoing management from age 18 had been discussed with the young person

▶ if transition was thought to be necessary, a transition planning meeting had been arranged

▶ the transition process had been started by contacting adult services.

Data analysis

The outcome measure was the proportion of cases compliant with each of the above points.

Resources required

People

This audit can be performed by a single doctor.

Time

This will depend on the number of patients in the service and the system in place to identify patients. In a service covering a population of 116 500, approximately 50 patients are likely to have ADHD, 10 of school-leaving age. Once the notes have been located, 1 day should be allowed for data collection, collation and write-up.

Results

The majority of CAMHS patients with ADHD who were of school-leaving age (and therefore should have begun transition planning according to the NICE guideline) did not have any documented transition planning. Those who had been discharged from the service mostly had a planned and agreed discharge and the vast majority would not have required transition planning.

Recommendations

▶ There should be discussion between adult services and CAMHS regarding previously agreed transition policy and the findings of this audit (e.g. at a clinical governance meeting).

▶ There should be clear written information for clinicians about what steps are required for transition and who (CAMHS or adult services) is responsible at each stage.

▶ There should be written information about adult services specifically for young people with ADHD and their parents.

Faraone, S. V., Biederman, J. & Mick, E. (2006) The age-dependent decline of attention deficit hyperactivity disorder: a meta-analysis of follow-up studies. *Psychological Medicine*, **36**, 159–165.

National Institute for Health and Clinical Excellence (2008) *Diagnosis and Management of ADHD in Children, Young People and Adults* (CG72). NICE. Available at http://guidance.nice.org.uk/CG72 (accessed October 2010).

Willoughby, M. T. (2003) Developmental course of ADHD symptomatology during the transition from childhood to adolescence: a review with recommendations. *Journal of Child Psychology and Psychiatry*, **44**, 88–106.

67. Violent incidents: management

Jenny Dale, Anupam Dharmadhikari, Anuprabha Wickramasinghe and Gabrielle Milner

Setting

The setting for this audit was a psychiatric high-dependency area in a general adult psychiatric in-patient unit. However, the audit could be replicated on any psychiatric in-patient facility.

Background

Acts of violence by patients, including assaults on staff, constitute a major management problem in psychiatric services. In 1999, the National Health Service (NHS) launched a zero tolerance campaign to reduce violence against its staff. However, violent incidents are still frequent in treatment settings and there is evidence that the incidence is increasing, particularly within mental health. Violence has significant physical, psychological and financial consequences – reportedly, violent incidents cost the NHS around £69 million a year, excluding the human cost. Safe and effective management of violence is important and is the topic of a guideline produced in 2005 by the National Institute for Health and Clinical Excellence (NICE).

Standards

The standards for the audit were derived from NICE guideline on the short-term management of disturbed/violent behaviour in in-patient psychiatric settings and emergency departments. The guidance is detailed and it would not be feasible to audit against all of the standards. The following were selected:

▶ There should be a comprehensive (and up-to-date) risk assessment/management plan.
▶ There should be evidence of the early use of de-escalation.
▶ Observations should be used to engage the patient positively.
▶ The use of physical interventions should occur only after de-escalation fails.
▶ Where physical restraint is used, vital signs should be monitored.
▶ There should be evidence of reassessment of the care plan after physical interventions.
▶ Incidents should be reported contemporaneously.

Method

Data collection

A data-collection tool (pro forma) was used to collect the following information:

▶ patient details – age, gender, ethnicity, date of admission, Mental Health Act status, diagnosis
▶ incident details – date, time, location, involvement of alcohol/drugs, observation levels, type of incident, presence of injury
▶ preventative measures – up-to-date risk assessment and management plan
▶ immediate management – use of de-escalation, rapid tranquillisation and physical restraint

▶ short-term management – incident reporting, clinical risk review, use of relevant resources.

Data were collected retrospectively in relation to a 12-month period for all the in-patients admitted to the unit. The incidents were identified and the incident reporting forms were examined. These should be easily accessible with the help of the ward clerk/ward manager. Some trusts may hold this information electronically. Patient records were screened for additional information.

Data analysis

The percentage of incidents meeting each of the standards was calculated. Expected compliance with the standards was 100%.

Resources required

People

It is recommended that two people collect the data. Multidisciplinary involvement may be appropriate. There was active involvement of the ward manager in the original audit.

Time

For an audit of 30 admissions with a total of 65 violent incidents, 2 weeks should be sufficient, depending on ease of availability of incident reporting forms and case notes.

Results

▶ Only a small group of patients were involved in the majority of the violent incidents.

▶ Staff were the primary targets in most incidents.

▶ De-escalation techniques were employed in only a minority of incidents.

▶ Rapid tranquillisation was the commonest modality of intervention to control the violent incidents.

▶ The incident forms were completed on the same day in nearly all of the instances.

Recommendations

▶ De-escalation should be rigorously promoted as a method of managing violent incidents.

▶ The importance of both physical health assessments and monitoring of vital signs in the management of acutely disturbed behaviour should be highlighted to staff.

▶ There should be regular staff training in the management of violent incidents.

National Institute for Health and Clinical Excellence (2005) *Violence: The Short-Term Management of Disturbed/Violent Behaviour in In-patient Settings and Emergency Departments* (CG25). NICE. Available at http://guidance.nice.org.uk/CG25 (accessed October 2010).

68. Waiting times

Ged Garry

Setting

Although this audit was specifically designed for a psychotherapy service, the principles could be applied to any setting where referrals are processed via a triage system that involves practitioners from different disciplines, such as community mental health teams or child and adolescent mental health services.

Background

In recent years there has been a move towards team working and referrals are more likely to be made to a service rather than a named individual. The way in which these referrals are processed varies. In the case of the specialist psychotherapy service, referrals were processed by clerical staff and forwarded to a referrals manager, who presented them at a weekly meeting of therapists from different psychotherapeutic disciplines (cognitive, psychodynamic, psychoanalytic, humanistic, etc.). The referrals were then allocated to what was considered to be the most appropriate modality. There was a perception within the team that this system was inefficient, resulting in undue delays to first assessment.

Standards

The service was benchmarked against the standard set in *The NHS Plan* (Department of Health, 2000) that no patient should wait longer than 13 weeks for a first appointment for non-urgent treatment. The interval between the receipt of a referral and its discussion at a referral meeting was also audited against a locally agreed standard of 1 week.

Method

Data collection
All referrals to the service in a calendar year were examined.

Data analysis
The number of referrals and the number and proportion of patients given appointments for assessment were calculated. Waiting times (defined as time from receipt of referral to date of first appointment offered) and time to discussion in the referrals meeting were also calculated.

The audit was repeated following implementation of an action plan (see below). Differences in the mean waiting times between the first audit and the second audit were then examined for statistical significance using an independent-samples t-test in SPSS version 12.0.

Resources required

People
The audit collected data on all referrals in a calendar year (more than 300 referrals) and was undertaken by two people. A less ambitious audit is recommended.

Time

With an efficient database it is estimated that data collection for 100 referrals would take no longer than 6 hours.

Results

An unacceptable number of patients were waiting longer than the 13-week standard. This was due in part to delays in referrals being discussed in the referrals meeting. Following the implementation of the action plan (see below) re-audit demonstrated a statistically significant improvement in waiting times.

Recommendations

The following action plan was implemented:

▶ Referrals meetings would be held no less than weekly (including holiday periods).

▶ Referrals meetings would prioritise the allocation of cases.

▶ Correspondence with referrers to seek additional information would be kept to a minimum. Ways of improving the quality of information provided by referrers would be explored.

▶ For each referral the 13-week deadline would be highlighted in the database.

▶ An up-to-date record of therapists' case-loads would be maintained.

▶ More flexible ways of working (such as uncoupling the assessment and treatment phases of therapy) would be promoted.

Department of Health (2000) *The NHS Plan: A Plan for Investment, A Plan for Reform*. The Stationery Office. Available at http://www.dh.gov.uk/en/Publicationsandstatistics/Publications/PublicationsPolicyAndGuidance/DH_4002960 (accessed October 2010).

VI. Training

Audits
Course attendance
Safety
Workplace-based assessments

69. Audits

Mark Lovell

Setting

This audit is relevant to all trainee psychiatrists and their trainers. It should be combined with training on the audit cycle.

Background

All doctors 'must take part in regular and systematic audit' (General Medical Council, 2006). Depending on where trainees are in their training, their knowledge, ability and motivation to partake in audit may vary. Demonstration of the understanding and principles of audit is one of the essential competencies that are required of an ST2 level trainee (Royal College of Psychiatrists, 2009). This audit allows a training scheme or trust to establish what proportion of its trainees are partaking in audit currently or recently, any reasons for not doing audit and the support that they have received from their trainers.

Standards

The four main audit standards for this audit were taken from the document *Specialist Training in Psychiatry* (Royal College of Psychiatrists, 2009):

▶ Trainees should undertake an audit in every placement.
▶ Trainees should endeavour to complete the audit cycle.
▶ Trainers should advise trainees about suitable audit projects or direct them to a nominated audit lead.
▶ Trainers should assist trainees in implementing changes suggested by audits.

Method

Data collection

Questionnaires were sent to all relevant psychiatric trainees either by post (with a return envelope) or by email. The following questions were asked:

1 Are you currently involved in audit activity?
2 If not currently, when were you last involved?
3 If not, why are you currently not involved in audit?
4 Have you ever completed the audit cycle?
5 If not, why has this not occurred?
6 Has your current trainer advised you on suitable audit projects or directed you to a nominated audit lead?
7 If you have previously completed an audit, did your trainer assist you in implementing changes suggested by your audit?

Data analysis

The replies for questions 1, 4, 6 and 7 were taken to represent the standards. This allowed a calculation of the compliance with the standard.

The replies to questions 2, 3 and 5 were qualitative and were used for discussion purposes and to guide recommendations.

Resources required

People

For a small group of trainee psychiatrists (e.g. within a hospital), this audit can be completed by one trainee. If the audit is to be completed for a larger group (e.g. multiple hospitals or a training scheme), one trainee per site would be recommended, to facilitate data collection and dissemination of the findings.

Time

This audit can be completed within 1 month, allowing for questionnaire returns and data analysis and write-up.

Results

The original audit found that not all trainees were currently involved in audit, nor did they all receive direct support from their trainers. Reasons cited were:

▶ not being aware that they had to do an audit in each post
▶ working towards professional examinations
▶ currently concentrating on other training needs.

The frequency of changing post for trainees meant that they generally started new audits rather than completing the cycle of a previous audit.

Recommendations

▶ It would be useful to create a register of current audit activity for all trainees. This might increase the amount of audit activity and the number of audit cycles completed.
▶ A regular training session should be held (every 6 months) on the audit cycle for new trainees and trainer involvement in the trainee audit process should be increased.
▶ With the support of trainers guiding trainees towards suitable audits, the quality and relevance of audits might improve, and rather than trainees simply completing audits for educational reasons, they could contribute to the clinical governance systems within a trust and thus improve services.

General Medical Council (2006) *Good Medical Practice*. GMC. Available at http://www.gmc-uk.org/guidance/good_medical_practice.asp (accessed October 2010).

Royal College of Psychiatrists (2009) *Specialist Training in Psychiatry* (OP69). RCPsych. Available at http://www.rcpsych.ac.uk/publications/collegereports/op/op69.aspx (accessed October 2010).

70. Course attendance

Greg Lydall

Setting

This audit may apply to all doctors within a hospital, directorate or trust.

Background

Ongoing training of staff, including doctors, in safety and other aspects of National Health Service (NHS) work is important for maintaining skills and knowledge. There is national and local policy on training requirements. The aim of this audit was to assess 12-monthly levels of compliance with mandatory and optional training according to national and trust policy using an online survey tool. It may be adapted to a paper-based survey.

Standards

Standards were obtained from a range of documents. Of particular relevance were the following standards for specific areas of medical practice:

▶ infection control requires annual training (Department of Health, 2008)
▶ basic life support requires annual training (Resuscitation Council, 2008)
▶ breakaway techniques requires training on starting employment and annually thereafter (Department of Health, 2005)
▶ the care programme approach (CPA) requires training on starting employment (Department of Health, 2001)
▶ child protection requires 1 day of training every 2 years for those working with children, or a half-day every 2 years for those not working with children (Chief Secretary to the Treasury, 2003).

NHS organisations are increasingly being audited by the Audit Commission regarding mandatory training. The target was that these standards were met for all doctors.

Method

Data collection

The medical staffing or medical education departments should have a list of email addresses for all doctors. Early liaison with the audit department and these departments is important.

Data were captured using an online survey tool piloted previously. Two rounds of emails were sent out to all doctors (at all grades) in the trust. Responding doctors were asked about basic demographic information (grade, site and months in post) and to answer yes or no to a list of courses that they might have attended in the past 12 months.

Reasons for not attending were asked about and could include:

▶ did not know about it
▶ did not want to
▶ not enough time
▶ some training seen as inappropriate.

Free-text responses were allowed.

Doctors were asked what might change to improve attendance. They could choose one or more of the following options:

- easier access and protected time
- multiple themes combined in a regular training session (e.g. weekly)
- reminders and deadlines via email
- improving the relevance of some courses
- improved access to e-learning.

Data analysis

The percentage of doctors answering yes in relation to each course was calculated, together with the response rate (number of responses/number of doctors.)

Resources required

People

It is suggested that one person working with the agreement of the medical staffing department is required.

Time

The total lenght of time needed for this audit was 8 hours.

Results

Doctors' attendance at mandatory and optional training was poor, and some staff groups performed below average. After the audit, the annual appraisal process for all doctors included an evaluation of mandatory training, and a re-audit 2 years later revealed marked improvement.

Recommendations

- A list of mandatory courses should feature in the corporate and site induction for all doctors.
- Mandatory courses should be promoted by articles in the trust email update, to increase awareness of them.
- The focus should initially be on improving mandatory attendance, through the following measures:
  - include the mandatory training list in annual appraisals for all doctors, and ensure that incomplete courses are re-checked at subsequent appraisals
  - consider how to secure protected time (as far as possible within a clinical setting) for mandatory training
  - increase the awareness of senior/consultant staff of the necessary courses.

Chief Secretary to the Treasury (2003) *Every Child Matters*. The Stationery Office.

Department of Health (2001) *An Audit Pack for Monitoring the Care Programme Approach*. DH. Available at http://www.dh.gov.uk/en/Publicationsandstatistics/Publications/PublicationsPolicyAndGuidance/DH_4008226 (accessed October 2010).

Department of Health (2005) *Promoting Safer and Therapeutic Services. Implementing the National Syllabus in Mental Health and Learning Disability Services*. DH. Available at http://www.nhsbsa.nhs.uk/SecurityManagement/Documents/psts_implementing_syllabus.pdf (accessed October 2010).

Department of Health (2008) *The Health and Social Care Act 2008: Code of Practice for the NHS on the Prevention and Control of Healthcare Associated Infections and Related Guidance*. DH. Available at http://www.dh.gov.uk/en/Publicationsandstatistics/Publications/PublicationsPolicyAndGuidance/DH_110288 (accessed October 2010).

Resuscitation Council (2008) *Standards for Clinical Practice and Training*. Resuscitation Council (UK).

71. Safety

Ollie White, Gautam Gulati and Ratna Ghosh

Setting

This audit is not service-specific and spans all directorates where psychiatric trainees work.

Background

Safety for psychiatric trainees is a key indicator in the quality assurance of a training scheme. This has repeatedly been emphasised as an important issue by the Royal College of Psychiatrists (1999, 2006, 2008) and in recent psychiatric literature (Dibben *et al*, 2008).

Standards

Standards were obtained from the Royal College of Psychiatrists' Council Report 134, *Safety for Psychiatrists* (2006). This augments the previous Royal College of Psychiatrists Council Report 78, *Safety for Trainees in Psychiatry* (1999). The following standards were of particular relevance:

▶ induction and safety training (e.g. de-escalation and breakaway)
▶ use of an alarm system
▶ lone-worker policy
▶ guidance/debriefing in the event of an assault
▶ environmental safety aspects of interview rooms (e.g. panic buttons, door opening outwards, inspection windows)
▶ safety of on-call accommodation.

Method

Data collection

As the above standards should be met for all trainees, it was necessary to identify all trainees within a programme. This can be done by contacting the relevant medical staffing department or medical education department.

A survey was developed with the aim of obtaining information directly from trainees about whether standards were being met, including the opportunity for trainees to comment about the reasons why standards were not met.

In order to obtain the highest possible response rate and ensure ease of distribution, a web-based survey tool was used. The survey could then be sent electronically to all trainees within the programme. Alternatively, postal questionnaires may be sent.

It is likely to be necessary to send email or written reminders to help ensure a high response rate.

Data analysis

Responses were analysed not only for the extent to which criteria were being met, but also for the stated reasons given by trainees as to why criteria were not met in their particular situations. Sub-analyses examined specific clinical situations where the meeting of standards varied. Examples included in-hours compared with out-of-hours working, and prison settings compared with out-patient settings.

Resources required

People

It is suggested that this audit is undertaken by at least two people, owing to the amount of information collected. At least one person should be reasonably competent with information technology if the survey is to be distributed online. Additional support from trainees with links to peer groups might be useful to aid distribution and increase response rates.

Time

For a training scheme with 70 trainees it is estimated that the data collection will take 12 hours. The time required for trainees to respond to the online survey needs to be considered (approximately 3–4 weeks).

Results

When this audit was conducted in two separate locations, a response rate of approximately 65% was obtained. Results revealed good environmental safety safeguards in in-patient areas but that focus should be given to improving out-patient and community settings, including out-of-hours assessment locations. Attendance at de-escalation and breakaway training was generally good but required further improvement.

Recommendations

▶ The audit findings should be discussed with the head of school, college tutors, training programme directors and directors of medical education.

▶ A collaborative plan should be agreed for improvement where necessary, including the development and modification of trust policies.

Dibben, C., O'Shea, R., Chang, R., et al (2008) Safety for psychiatrists – from trainee to consultant. *Psychiatric Bulletin*, **32**, 85–87.

Royal College of Psychiatrists (1999) *Safety for Trainees in Psychiatry* (CR78). RCPsych. Available at http://www.rcpsych.ac.uk/pdf/cr78.pdf (accessed October 2010).

Royal College of Psychiatrists (2006) *Safety for Psychiatrists* (CR134). RCPsych. Available at http://www.rcpsych.ac.uk/publications/collegereports/cr/cr134.aspx (accessed October 2010).

Royal College of Psychiatrists (2008) *Postgraduate Training in Psychiatry: Essential Information for Trainees and Trainers* (OP65). RCPsych. Available at http://www.rcpsych.ac.uk/files/pdfversion/OP65.pdf (accessed October 2010).

72. Workplace-based assessments

Lorraine Pauley

Setting

This audit is relevant to all trainee psychiatrists undertaking workplace-based assessments (WPBAs) as part of their ongoing training and to those involved in conducting assessments.

Background

In 2007 WPBAs were introduced to medical training in the UK as a means of facilitating regular and robust assessment of trainees, both formatively and summatively. The aim of the audit was to evaluate trainee experiences of WPBAs and to determine whether current standards were being met.

Standards

Current standards for WPBAs were compiled from existing guidelines documented by the Royal College of Psychiatrists (2007*a–c*), the Postgraduate Medical Education and Training Board (PMETB) (2005) and the Department of Health (2007). In summary, these were as follows:

▶ A meeting should be arranged between the trainee and the educational supervisor for an initial educational appraisal, preferably in the first week of the placement. Trainees should be helped to draw up a personal development plan, including the planning of WPBAs.

▶ Trainees should plan which WPBAs they need to complete in each placement and discuss them with their educational supervisor.

▶ The educational supervisor's role is to advise and encourage trainees to develop their competencies and to demonstrate this through their participation in regular assessments.

▶ Trainees should not be assessed solely by the educational supervisor. Evidence must be triangulated whenever possible (i.e. it must be provided by different assessors, on different occasions and if possible using different methods).

▶ The trainee is responsible for organising the assessments.

▶ If a patient is involved in a WPBA, his or her agreement to participate should be sought in advance.

▶ The trainee should have WPBAs completed regularly throughout the placement to demonstrate effective review and appraisal.

All trainees should be able to meet all of the current standards for WPBAs.

Method

Data collection

A questionnaire was devised based on the compiled standards, allowing each standard to be evaluated individually. Space was provided alongside each question to allow trainees to make additional comments. The questionnaire could be distributed to all trainees currently working within a deanery, training programme or trust.

Data analysis

For each standard, the percentage of trainees who were able to meet the standard was calculated. Additional comments made by trainees provided qualitative information.

Resources required

People

This audit can be conducted by one person (for about 80 trainees) but may require an additional person if there is a larger number of questionnaires to be evaluated.

Time

Trainees may be sent the questionnaire by email after completion of the Annual Review of Competence Progression (ARCP) and given up to 4 weeks to respond. Reminders should be sent during this time. Paper-based surveys may also be used.

Results

Completed questionnaires were received from 34 of 81 trainees sent a copy (42%). Nearly two-thirds (59%) of trainees had difficulty accessing appropriate assessors. Only two of the standards gained total compliance:

- ▶ all trainees met with their educational supervisor at the start of their first placement
- ▶ all trainees completed the required number of WPBAs.

Recommendations

- ▶ Improvements should be made to the guidance available for potential assessors.
- ▶ A re-audit should be done after the next ARCP process.

Department of Health (2007) *Guide to Postgraduate Specialty Training in the UK (Gold Guide)* (1st edition). DH. Available at http://www.jrcptb.org.uk/SiteCollectionDocuments/Gold%20Guide.pdf (accessed October 2010).

Postgraduate Medical Education and Training Board (2005) *Workplace Based Assessment – A Paper from the PMETB Workplace Based Assessment Subcommittee*. PMETB.

Royal College of Psychiatrists (2007a) *Educational Supervisors' Guide to Workplace Based Assessment and Appraisal of Psychiatric Trainees*. RCPsych. Available at https://training.rcpsych.ac.uk/educational-supervisors%E2%80%99-guide-workplace-based-assessment-and-appraisal-psychiatric-trainees (accessed October 2010).

Royal College of Psychiatrists (2007b) *The RCPsych Brief Guide to the Curriculum and Assessment System for Psychiatry Specialty Training*. London: Royal College of Psychiatrists. Available at http://www.rcpsych.ac.uk/docs/Briefguide.doc (accessed October 2010).

Royal College of Psychiatrists (2007c) *Trainees' Guide to Workplace Based Assessments*. London: Royal College of Psychiatrists. Available at http://www.rcpsych.ac.uk/.../Trainees%20guide%20to%20WPBA%2031%2010%2007.doc (accessed October 2010).

VII. Treatment

73. Alcohol withdrawal: management

Jim Bolton, Siobhan Quinn, Rani Samuel, Borislav Iankov and Anna Stout

Setting

This audit may be particularly relevant to liaison psychiatry services involved in the management of patients with alcohol dependency in the general hospital setting. It may also be relevant to mental health in-patient units managing patients in alcohol withdrawal.

Background

Poorly managed alcohol detoxification can cause distress to individuals and their carers, and increase referral rates to liaison psychiatry services. Individuals who have undergone inadequate detoxification are less likely to engage in subsequent alcohol rehabilitation. Thiamine deficiency secondary to alcohol dependency can lead to permanent neurological damage such as Wernicke–Korsakoff syndrome. Appropriate alcohol detoxification and vitamin prophylaxis are crucial in preventing these problems.

Standards

Standards were obtained from guidelines for the pharmacological management of alcohol withdrawal published by the Royal College of Physicians (2001) and the British Association for Psychopharmacology (Lingford-Hughes *et al*, 2004). The hospital guidelines derived from these documents are detailed in Appendix 2 to this book.

▶ For alcohol detoxification, prescriptions were judged to meet the standard if either chlordiazepoxide or diazepam was prescribed as a reducing regimen for an adequate duration.

▶ For vitamin prophylaxis, prescriptions met the standard if the dose, route and duration were in accordance with the guidelines.

Method

Data collection

For the duration of the audit, members of the general hospital liaison psychiatry team visited the acute admission wards daily to identify patients who had been prescribed an alcohol detoxification regime by the admitting medical or surgical team. Ward staff and hospital pharmacists cooperated in identifying such patients. Individual patients' prescription charts were assessed against the standards. In the first audit cycle, 27 prescription charts were scrutinised. Following a period of intervention, a second audit cycle scrutinised a further 22 prescription charts.

Data analysis

For each audit cycle, the percentage of charts where the prescription was judged to be in accordance with the guidelines was calculated for:

▶ alcohol detoxification
▶ vitamin prophylaxis.

Resources required

People

It is suggested that this audit is undertaken by at least two people, owing to the amount of information collected and the possible need to confer over cases where the adequacy of the prescription is unclear.

Time

For one audit cycle scrutinising 20–25 prescription charts, it is estimated that the data collection would take 15 hours.

Results

▶ In the first audit cycle, 48% of prescription charts met the standard for detoxification. In the second cycle, 91% met the standard, an increase of 43 percentage points.

▶ The standard for vitamin prophylaxis was met in 19% of cases in the first audit cycle and in 82% in the second cycle, an increase of 63 percentage points.

Recommendations

The following interventions were undertaken following the first audit cycle:

▶ A written prescribing protocol, based upon national guidelines and adapted in discussion with the hospital pharmacists, was compiled and distributed in the general hospital.

▶ The protocol was published in the hospital's handbook of medical emergencies issued to junior doctors.

▶ The protocol was also printed on laminated sheets and placed at visible sites on all medical and surgical wards.

▶ The protocol was included in teaching sessions on alcohol provided for junior doctors by the liaison psychiatry team.

A more detailed description of the audit and the guidelines created was compiled for publication (Quinn *et al*, 2008).

Lingford-Hughes, A. R., Welch, S. J. & Nutt, D. J. (2004) Evidence based guidelines for the pharmacological management of substance misuse, addiction and comorbidity: recommendations from the British Association for Psychopharmacology. *Journal of Psychopharmacology*, **18**, 293–335.

Quinn, S., Samuel, R., Bolton, J., *et al* (2008) Pharmacological management of alcohol withdrawal in a general hospital. *Psychiatric Bulletin*, **32**, 452–454.

Royal College of Physicians (2001) *Report of a Working Party: Alcohol – Can the NHS Afford It? Recommendations for a Coherent Alcohol Strategy for Hospitals*. RCP.

74. Anticholinesterase inhibitors: monitoring of cardiac side-effects

Larissa Ryan

Setting

This audit is designed to be carried out within the setting of an out-patient memory clinic in old age psychiatry.

Background

Acetylcholinesterase inhibitors are licensed and widely used for the treatment of dementia. There is a potential for cardiac side-effects from these medications, particularly in the elderly population. This is due to their cholinergic effect, acting to slow the heart rate down by enhancing vagal activity. This bradycardiac effect has led to concerns about serious arrhythmias or heart block, but could also lead to pre-syncope due to a slow pulse. Dizziness leading to falls in older people could have serious consequences, such as fractures or intracranial bleeds. Rowland *et al* (2007) addressed this issue of cardiac complications in a review of randomised controlled trials of the three cholinesterase inhibitors, and recommended that a minimal level of cardiac monitoring is suitable.

Standards

Standards were taken from a protocol suggested by Rowland *et al* (2007) and were as follows:

▶ All patients considered for treatment with cholinesterase inhibitors in the memory clinic should have a symptom enquiry and pulse check at baseline.

▶ All patients currently on treatment with cholinesterase inhibitors in the memory clinic should have a symptom enquiry and pulse check at each 6-monthly follow-up visit.

Method

Data collection

A report was generated showing all patients seen in a memory clinic over a defined period. This could be obtained from a computer system or clinic records. Patients were included in the audit only if they were currently receiving treatment with cholinesterase inhibitors, or were due to start such treatment. The medical notes for these patients were then obtained and analysed.

For all patients already on a cholinesterase inhibitor (and those due to start treatment with one), the presence in the notes of the following was recorded:

▶ demographic details

▶ presence or absence of any pre-existing cardiac disease

▶ previous treatment with a rate-altering medication, other than cholinesterase inhibitors

▶ the presence or absence of symptoms of dizziness, syncope, falls or 'funny turns'

▶ a pulse rate check.

In addition, for patients already on a cholinesterase inhibitor, the notes were checked for documentation of which medication they were on, its dose and duration of treatment.

Data analysis

The following were calculated:

- percentage of patients with pre-existing cardiac disease
- percentage of patients previously on a rate-altering medication
- percentage of patients with documentation of a symptom enquiry
- percentage of patients with documentation of a pulse check.

Resources required

People

This audit could be carried out by one or two people (e.g. a psychiatrist and a memory clinic nurse).

Time

For a sample size of 50 patients it is estimated that data collection would take 10–12 hours.

Results

A significant proportion of patients seen had pre-existing cardiac disease and a lesser proportion were already being treated with cardiac rate-altering medication other than cholinesterase inhibitors. There was poor performance on documentation of pre-existing cardiac disease and relevant medications, and also on documentation of symptom enquiries and pulse rate checks.

Recommendations

- The audit results should be made available to clinicians working in the memory clinic, with the aim of promoting good practice by increasing knowledge of this area.
- A brief pro forma should be designed, with tick boxes for symptoms and a space to record the pulse rate; the pro forma could be completed by any member of the multidisciplinary team.
- The audit should be repeated in 6 months.

Rowland, J. P., Rigby, J., Harper, A. C., *et al* (2007) Cardiovascular monitoring with acetylcholinesterase inhibitors: a clinical protocol. *Advances in Psychiatric Treatment*, 13, 178–184.

75. Anticholinesterase inhibitors: prescribing

Felicity Richards

Setting

This audit is relevant to psychiatrists working in the field of old age psychiatry. It can relate to either in-patient or out-patient settings, but would be of particular relevance to memory clinics.

Background

Anti-dementia medications are not without significant side-effects, and close monitoring is necessary to ensure that anticholinesterase (AchE) inhibitors are being used appropriately. In November 2006, the National Institute for Health and Clinical Excellence (NICE) revised its guideline on prescribing and monitoring the use of AchE inhibitors (donepezil, rivastigmine, galantamine and memantine) in Alzheimer's dementia. These guidelines limited the use of these medications to patients with moderate Alzheimer's disease, defined as those with scores of 10–20 (out of 30) on the Mini-Mental State Examination (MMSE) (Folstein *et al*, 1975).

Standards

Standards were obtained from the NICE (2006) guideline on prescribing and monitoring the use of AchE inhibitors. Of particular relevance were:

▶ Medications can be prescribed only by specialists in elderly care (psychiatrists, neurologists and physicians specialising in care of the elderly) for patients with an MMSE score between 10 and 20.
▶ Carers' views should be sought at baseline.
▶ Patients who continue the drug should be reviewed at 6-monthly intervals by means of MMSE score, along with a global, functional and behavioural assessment.
▶ Carers' views should be sought regarding the patient's condition at follow-up.
▶ The drugs should be continued only while the patient's MMSE score remains at or above 10 points and his or her global, functional and behavioural condition remains at a level where the drug is considered to be having a worthwhile effect.
▶ Prescribing can occur outside these guidelines, but clear documentation outlining these clinical decisions is necessary.

Method

Data collection

The medical notes of patients who had been in the service since November 2006 and who were currently prescribed AchE inhibitors were selected. Notes were examined to ascertain documented evidence of the following:

▶ type of dementia diagnosed (Alzheimer's disease, mixed-type, vascular, etc.)

- the clinician who initiated treatment
- type of medication begun (i.e. donepezil, galantamine or rivastigmine)
- baseline recordings of MMSE score, carers' views and assessments of functioning
- frequency of follow up, evidence of ongoing MMSE assessment, carers' views and assessments of the patient's global, functional and behavioural condition
- reasons for discontinuation of treatment such as side-effects, MMSE score falling below 10, deterioration while on medication
- clear documentation to support clinical decisions that vary from the guidance.

Data analysis

The percentage of assessments with the above evidence recorded in the medical notes was calculated. The aim was for 100% compliance with the standards.

Resources required

People

Two people were needed to review approximately 50 case notes. This audit lends itself to multidisciplinary involvement.

Time

For at least 50 sets of case notes, at least 2 working days should be allotted to this audit.

Results

This audit illustrated that AchE inhibitors continued to be prescribed for mild dementia and highlighted difficulties in the implementation of the new guidance. This may reflect the varying opinions of clinicians regarding the use of guidelines and also the perceived efficacy of the treatments.

Recommendations

- The NICE guideline does allow prescribing in mild Alzheimer's disease, under certain circumstances, and the importance of adequate documentation for these cases should be highlighted.
- If a patient is unable to complete an MMSE (e.g. a patient is too anxious, has dysphasia, or the dementia is too severe), this should be clearly documented.
- Reasons should be given in the case notes for continuing AchE inhibitors if the MMSE score has fallen for non-cognitive (behavioural or psychological) symptoms associated with dementia.
- An 'anti-dementia drug record sheet' should be used.
- An 'activities of daily living' questionnaire could be sent out with the initial appointment letter for carers to complete.

Folstein, M. F., Folstein, S. E., McHugh, P. R., et al (1975) 'Mini-mental state'. A practical method for grading the cognitive state of patients for the clinician. Journal of Psychiatric Research, 12, 189–198.

National Institute for Health and Clinical Excellence (2006) Donepezil, Galantamine, Rivastigmine (Review) and Memantine for the Treatment of Alzheimer's Disease. NICE. Available at http://www.nice.org.uk/TA111 (accessed October 2010).

76. Antimuscarinic medications

Rohit Bhardwaj and Sandip Deshpande

Setting

This audit has relevance across all settings where antimuscarinic medications are prescribed (e.g. acute in-patient, rehabilitation and community settings).

Background

Antimuscarinic drugs are extensively used in mental health settings. However, clinical research and guidance on their use are scant. Their longer-term side-effects include autonomic effects, cognitive impairment, agitation and the initiation or worsening of tardive dyskinesia (Birmingham *et al*, 1999). Hence, clinicians need regularly to monitor the use of these medications (World Health Organization, 1990).

Standards

Standards were developed from several evidence-based sources (Birmingham *et al*, 1999; Steele, 2000; Taylor *et al*, 2007; Joint Formulary Committee, 2009):

▶ Only one antimuscarinic should be prescribed for each patient.

▶ Doses of antimuscarinics should not exceed the limits set out in the *British National Formulary* (*BNF*) (Joint Formulary Committee, 2009).

▶ Continued use of antimuscarinics should be reviewed at least every 3 months.

▶ If on antimuscarinics for more than 3 months, dose reduction should be attempted in the absence of extra-pyramidal side-effects.

▶ Antimuscarinic use on an 'as required' (p.r.n. basis) should be reviewed at least once every 4 weeks.

▶ Antimuscarinic drug prescriptions should be removed from the p.r.n. chart if the drug has not been administered in the previous 2 months.

The target is that these standards are met for all patients who are prescribed antimuscarinic medication.

Method

Data collection

Current prescription data (either drug cards or last clinic letter) and the medical notes on antimuscarinic medication were examined for each patient in the relevant service of interest. Patients who were currently prescribed anti-muscarinics were included in the audit, with a view to obtaining the following information:

▶ the number of in-patients on antimuscarinic medication and their diagnoses

▶ details of antipsychotic medications, including names, whether typical or atypical and number

▶ frequency of antimuscarinic use, their number, names, whether their total dose exceeded *BNF* limits and duration of use

▶ whether dose reduction or withdrawal had been considered or attempted where appropriate, for patients on antimuscarinics for more than 3 or 2 months, respectively

▶ whether prescribed p.r.n. antimuscarinic medication had been reviewed within the preceding month

▶ total time on the current dose of antimuscarinic medication.

Data analysis
Data can be analysed at the level of the trust/health board, or between teams in order to compare practice across an organisation, via the percentage of the patient sample for whom each standard was met.

Resources required
People
The audit requires a minimum of one person to collect data for each site across a trust.

Time
It is estimated that data collection would take about 10 minutes for each patient on antimuscarinic medication.

Results
▶ Of 219 in-patients audited, 102 were prescribed antimuscarinic medication.

▶ Only one agent was used for each patient. Procyclidine was the most commonly used.

▶ The prescribed dose of antimuscarinic medication exceeded *BNF* limits for seven patients.

▶ Over half (53%) of the in-patients were on regular antimuscarinic medication for more than 3 months.

▶ Prescriptions of antimuscarinics were not reviewed as regularly as suggested.

Recommendations
▶ Organisational guidance and protocols should be developed on antimuscarinic use, with a view to improving review of prescribing practices and clinical documentation

Birmingham, L., McClelland, N. & Bradley, C. (1999) Role of PRN antimuscarinic medication in the treatment of antipsychotic-induced extrapyramidal movement disorders. *Psychiatric Bulletin*, 23, 368–369.

Joint Formulary Committee (2009) *British National Formulary* (58th edition). British Medical Association & Royal Pharmaceutical Society of Great Britain.

Steele, J. (2000) An audit of anti-muscarinic drug use at the state hospital. *Psychiatric Bulletin*, 24, 61–64.

Taylor, D., Paton, C. & Kerwin, R. (2007) *The Maudsley Prescribing Guidelines* (9th edition). Informa Healthcare.

World Health Organization (1990) Prophylactic use of anticholinergics in patients on long term neuroleptic treatment. A consensus statement. *British Journal of Psychiatry*, 156, 412.

77. Antipsychotics: combined and high dose

Amber Shingleton-Smith, Carol Paton and Thomas Barnes

Setting

This audit is relevant to many psychiatric services, but particularly to adult in-patient wards.

Background

The use of antipsychotic medication in combination or at high dose – defined as exceeding the maximum dose recommended in the *British National Formulary* (*BNF*) (Joint Formulary Committee, 2009) – has been relatively consistent over time, despite the existence of evidence-based, national guidance advising against such practice. Neither the effectiveness nor the side-effect burden associated with this approach has been studied systematically in clinical trials. The evidence that does exist suggests that the potential for harm may outweigh the potential for benefit.

This audit was designed as part of a quality improvement programme from the Prescribing Observatory of Mental Health (POMH-UK; see http://www.rcpsych.ac.uk/pomh) on the prescription of high-dose and combined antipsychotics on adult acute and intensive-care wards.

Standards

The standards were derived from the schizophrenia guideline produced by the National Institute for Health and Clinical Excellence, as updated in 2009, and the Royal College of Psychiatrists' 2006 *Consensus Statement on High Dose Antipsychotic Medication*.

- ▶ The dose of an individual antipsychotic should be within its *BNF* limits A 'high dose' of antipsychotic is defined here as a total daily dose (whether of a single antipsychotic or combined antipsychotics) greater than the maximum recommended daily dose.
- ▶ Individuals receive only one antipsychotic at a time (with the exception of individuals with schizophrenia who are receiving clozapine but who have not responded sufficiently; and individuals who are changing from one antipsychotic to another).
- ▶ First- (typical) and second-generation (atypical) antipsychotic drugs are not prescribed concurrently (unless 'Any concurrent prescriptions are for a short period to cover changeover of medication', and 'Local teams should agree on what constitutes a changeover period for audit purposes').

Method

Data collection

Each participating mental health trust was invited to include as many acute adult admission and psychiatric intensive-care units as it wished. Teams were asked to submit data for all patients who, on a census day, occupied a bed on the selected wards and were being prescribed one or more antipsychotic drugs. The clinical records of these patients were examined for documentation of the following:

- demographic variables (age, gender, ethnicity)
- clinical variables (diagnostic grouping, Mental Health Act status)
- the names and dosage of all regular and p.r.n. antipsychotic drugs prescribed on the census day.

For each patient prescribed more than one antipsychotic, discussion with the responsible clinical team established the primary reason (i.e. clinical indication) for the combination. For these anonymised data, submission from each trust was via a web-based form and a secure web system to POMH-UK for analysis.

Data analysis

Data were analysed at national, trust and ward levels. Individualised reports on the proportion of patients for whom the standards were met were produced for participating trusts, to allow confidential benchmarking of prescribing practice in relation to other clinical teams within each trust, between trusts and against the total national sample.

Resources required

People

A local multidisciplinary team is required to organise data collection and to disseminate the findings within the trust.

Time

This will depend on the number of clinical teams taking part and cases entered, but each audit data-collection form should not take more than 10 minutes to complete and submit.

Results

A high proportion of acute, adult, psychiatric in-patients are prescribed a high dose of antipsychotic medication, and the use of combined antipsychotics and p.r.n. antipsychotic medication made a major contribution to this. At 12-month re-audit, there was little evidence of any change in prescribing practice. A supplementary audit was conducted a year later, and the majority of trusts that participated at all three stages of data collection showed substantial improvements against the audit standards over this longer time period.

Recommendations

A number of change interventions for trusts have been produced by POMH-UK aimed at raising awareness of the issues associated with prescribing combined and high-dose antipsychotics. The most powerful intervention has been the benchmarked audit data, presented in customised reports and slide sets.

Joint Formulary Committee (2009) *British National Formulary* (58th edition). British Medical Association & Royal Pharmaceutical Society of Great Britain.

National Institute for Health and Clinical Excellence (2009) *Schizophrenia: Core Interventions in the Treatment and Management of Schizophrenia in Primary and Secondary Care* (CG82). NICE. Available at http://guidance.nice.org.uk/CG82 (accessed October 2010).

Royal College of Psychiatrists (2006) *Revised Consensus Statement on High Dose Antipsychotic Medication* (CR138). RCPsych. Available at http://www.rcpsych.ac.uk/files/pdfversion/CR138.pdf (accessed October 2010).

78. Antipsychotics: prescribing

Madhusudan Deepak Thalitaya and Deepthi Gunatilake

Setting

This audit is relevant in any service where a high proportion of patients are likely to be prescribed antipsychotic medication.

Background

Guidelines on antipsychotic medication produced by the National Institute for Health and Clinical Excellence (NICE) suggests that atypical antipsychotics are preferred to typical antipsychotics because of their lesser side-effect profile and higher propensity for compliance. National Health Service trusts have an obligation to ensure that appropriate atypical drugs with the lowest purchase costs are considered before a prescription is made.

Standards

Standards were obtained from National Institute for Health and Clinical Excellence 2009 guidance on the use of atypical antipsychotic medication in schizophrenia. Of particular relevance are the following:

- The choice of antipsychotic medication should be made jointly by the prescriber and the (properly informed) patient and/or carer.
- Second-generation antipsychotics should be considered as the first-line treatment.
- Second-generation antipsychotics should be considered for patients who show or report unacceptable adverse effects caused by first-generation agents.
- Clozapine should be considered if the patient is unresponsive to two different antipsychotic medications (at least one being a second-generation antipsychotic).
- Depot medication should be used where there are grounds to suspect that a patient may be unlikely to adhere to prescribed oral therapy.
- The drug with the lowest purchase cost should be prescribed.
- Advance directives regarding patients' preference for treatment should be developed and documented.
- A comprehensive package of care should be considered.
- Second-generation antipsychotics and first-generation antipsychotics should not be prescribed together except during a changeover of medication.
- Justify reasons for dosages outside the range given in the *BNF* (Joint Formulary Committee, 2009).

Method

Data collection

A retrospective review of case notes and medication cards from all in-patients was used. It was helpful to use an audit pro forma based on the above standards.

Data analysis

The total percentage compliance with all the above standards was analysed using a computerised statistical package.

Resources required

People

This audit was conducted by two people to cover the entire in-patient population as well as to minimise bias.

Time

If data are collected by two clinicians, it is anticipated that no more than 6 hours will be required for this, and a further 4 hours for analysis and presentation.

Results

- ▶ Nearly three-quarters of the patients were on antipsychotic medication.
- ▶ Risperidone was the most commonly prescribed medication.
- ▶ All prescriptions were within the limits specified in the *BNF*.
- ▶ The audit revealed that the standards were achieved in all aspects except cost.
- ▶ There was limited documentation of the fact that consideration had been given to the cost of the medication before prescribing.
- ▶ The documentation of discussions about treatment, capacity and consent was generally good.

Recommendations

- ▶ Clinical prescribing staff should ensure that decisions regarding choice of medication are made jointly with the patient and/or carer.
- ▶ If a patient has been transferred from another locality with medication, doctors should aim to discuss the indications and need for medication with the patient and carer and record these in the clinical notes.
- ▶ Clinicians should familiarise themselves with the cost of and recommended dose of each antipsychotic.
- ▶ Formulating a checklist to ensure compliance with the guidelines could be an option.

Joint Formulary Committee (2009) *British National Formulary* (58th edition). British Medical Association & Royal Pharmaceutical Society of Great Britain.

National Institute for Health and Clinical Excellence (2009) *Schizophrenia: Core Interventions in the Treatment and Management of Schizophrenia in Primary and Secondary Care* (CG82). NICE. Available at http://guidance.nice.org.uk/CG82 (accessed October 2010).

79. Antipsychotics: use in dementia

Vinay Sudhindra Rao and Judy Rubinsztein

Setting

This audit is particularly useful in old age psychiatry. Patients could be selected from in-patient and out-patient settings.

Background

Around 800 000 people in the UK have dementia, of whom 80% will be expected to have behavioural changes or psychological symptoms in the course of their illness (Overshott & Burns, 2005). The three main types of difficult-to-manage behaviours are associated with:

▶ agitation/aggression
▶ psychosis
▶ mood disorder.

The National Institute for Health and Clinical Excellence (NICE) (2006) and the *Drug and Therapeutics Bulletin* (2007) have published guidelines on the treatment of behavioural problems in patients with dementia. However, there are no medications currently licensed in the UK for these indications.

Standards

Based on the above guidance, the following standards were obtained:

▶ If patients are prescribed an antipsychotic medication, there should be documentation of their severe distress or of immediate risk of harm to themselves or others.
▶ Before a patient is started on or switched to an antipsychotic medication, there is documentation of the fact that the prescriber has considered important comorbid conditions such as cerebrovascular disease, diabetes mellitus, Parkinson's disease and hypercholesterolaemia.
▶ Discussion with the patient and/or carer is documented of the rationale behind starting on or switching to an antipsychotic medication, as well as discussion of its side-effects.

Method

Data collection

A list was obtained of all patients seen by older people's mental health services within the stipulated time frame for the audit. From this, those who were diagnosed with dementia were shortlisted, and those who were started on or switched to an antipsychotic medication were identified. All documentation (hand-written, computerised and printed) was examined.

Data analysis

The proportion of case notes with appropriate documentation was noted. A standard of 100% was set. A computerised database was used to tabulate and analyse the data.

Resources required

People

It is advisable to involve at least two people for the data collection, especially where there are large numbers of case notes involved.

Time

Data collection can be a time-consuming task when examining case notes.

Results

Among 307 patients screened, only eight were started on or switched to an antipsychotic medication within the audit duration of 2 months. Quetiapine was the preferred antipsychotic. Documentation was reasonably good, although 100% compliance was not achieved.

This audit raises awareness among clinicians of:

▶ the newly defined relatively increased risks of stroke and mortality related to prescribing all antipsychotic medications for behavioural problems in dementia

▶ the need to consider non-drug interventions first for patients with behavioural problems and the importance of considering medical comorbidity

▶ the need to use antipsychotics for patients only when they are severely distressed or at risk of harm to themselves or others

▶ the need to discuss the risks of all side-effects when starting antipsychotic medications with patients and/or their carers

▶ the importance of documentation.

Recommendations

▶ The trust should develop a protocol on this topic.

▶ The protocol could be incorporated in staff training.

▶ The audit should be repeated on a larger sample, to complete the audit cycle.

Drug and Therapeutics Bulletin (2007) How safe are antipsychotics in dementia. *Drug and Therapeutics Bulletin*, **45**, 81–85.

National Institute for Health and Clinical Excellence (2006) *Dementia: Supporting People with Dementia and Their Carers in Health and Social Care* (CG42). NICE. Available at http://www.nice.org.uk/nicemedia/pdf/CG042NICEGuideline.pdf (accessed October 2010).

Overshott, R. & Burns, A. (2005) Treatment of dementia. *Journal of Neurology, Neurosurgery and Psychiatry*, **76** (suppl. V), 53–59.

80. Attention-deficit hyperactivity disorder: prescribing

Matthew Impey

Setting

This audit is intended for a child and adolescent mental health service (CAMHS) involved in the initiation and monitoring of medications prescribed for attention-deficit hyperactivity disorder (ADHD).

Background

The diagnosis of ADHD is frequently made but still controversial. In children, it involves difficulties with concentration, excessive motor activity and impulsivity in a variety of environments (National Institute for Health and Clinical Excellence, 2008). Alongside behavioural interventions, medications are an important form of treatment and can be taken as short- or long-acting preparations. First-line treatments are stimulants (methylphenidate or dexamfetamine) or atomoxetine.

Standards

Audit criteria were based upon the National Institute for Health and Clinical Excellence's Technology Appraisal 98, *Methylphenidate, Atomoxetine and Dexamfetamine for ADHD in Children and Adolescents* (2006). This document looks specifically at ADHD medications. The target for meeting all standards was 100%.

▶ Drug treatments in ADHD are initiated by an appropriately qualified healthcare professional with expertise in ADHD. (In our locality, this could be either a CAMHS consultant or a paediatrician with specialist experience. In other regions, specialist nurses or pharmacists may also be able to initiate these medications.)

▶ Drug treatment is based on a comprehensive assessment and diagnosis. This was taken to require at least three assessments and use of a common rating questionnaire, for example the Conner's rating scale.

▶ Where drug treatment is appropriate, methylphenidate, atomoxetine or dexamfetamine is offered.

▶ The decision regarding choice of product considers:
  ▷ the presence of comorbid conditions
  ▷ adverse effects
  ▷ specific compliance issues
  ▷ the potential for drug diversion or misuse (stimulant medications are controlled substances and could be used illicitly by the patient or others)
  ▷ preferences of the child and parents or guardians.

Method

Data collection

Prescribing information was taken from multidisciplinary case notes from two sites. The sample included all the available notes (a total of 48 patients).

Data analysis

Outcomes were defined by how closely the standard met the target for completion. Comparisons were descriptive rather than statistical.

Resources required

People

The data could be collected by one person. If multiple sites are used, local collection can be performed by different individuals and later analysed as a whole.

Time

Data collection can take place over any period of time.

Results

- All medications were initiated by an appropriate healthcare professional.
- A comprehensive assessment took place in most cases, including use of Conner's scales in 78%.
- All patients were offered prescriptions of methylphenidate, dexamfetamine or atomoxetine. In general, consideration of comorbidity, adverse effects and patient/parent preferences were poorly recorded.
- Compliance issues and drug diversion were not considered in any cases, possibly because they were seen as very patient specific.
- There were some notable inter-site variations, with one location providing more comprehensive assessments and also considering patient preferences more frequently than the other.

Recommendations

- A form was developed to record important aspects of diagnosis and treatment. The design incorporated the above standards for comprehensive assessment, and also prompted clinicians to consider their medication choices in more detail.
- Re-audit was recommended for 1–2 years later, to allow a new set of patients to build up.
- At the point of re-audit, criteria can be taken from the full ADHD guidance issued by the National Institute for Health and Clinical Excellence (2008) following the completion of this audit.

National Institute for Health and Clinical Excellence (2006) *Methylphenidate, Atomoxetine and Dexamfetamine for Attention Deficit Hyperactivity Disorder (ADHD) in Children and Adolescents* (TA098). NICE. Available at http://www.nice.org.uk/nicemedia/pdf/TA098publicinfo.pdf (accessed October 2010).

National Institute for Health and Clinical Excellence (2008) *Attention Deficit Hyperactivity Disorder: Diagnosis and Management of ADHD in Children, Young People and Adults* (CG72). NICE. Available at http://guidance.nice.org.uk/CG72 (accessed October 2010).

81. Atypical antipsychotics: monitoring

Padma Suresh Babu

Setting

This audit is of relevance to all in-patient and out-patient settings. It was originally conducted in an in-patient child and adolescent intellectual disability setting.

Background

Antipsychotics are widely used for severe psychiatric disorders and for managing aggressive behaviours and anxiety related to autism. First-generation antipsychotics, while considered effective, are associated with serious acute and chronic side-effects that frequently limit their use. Second-generation antipsychotics are considered to be equally effective and are sometimes better tolerated. However, these newer antipsychotics are associated with metabolic side-effects, such as weight gain, hyperglycaemia, new-onset diabetes and dyslipidaemia. As these metabolic side-effects are so closely associated with the development of cardiovascular disease, monitoring and early intervention are crucial.

Standards

Standards were taken from the Maudsley guidelines (Taylor *et al*, 2007), which advise on recommended monitoring requirements for second-generation antipsychotic medication at baseline and follow-up:

▶ Baseline assessment should include full-blood count, and determination of HbA1c, urea and electrolytes, fasting lipid and fasting glucose levels, liver function tests, weight and blood pressure.

▶ Specific drugs require additional baseline tests:
  ▷ serum prolactin for amisulpride, olanzapine, risperidone and zotepine
  ▷ electrocardiography (ECG) for clozapine and zotepine
  ▷ thyroid function tests for quetiapine.

▶ Assessment after 6–12 months should include full blood count, and determination of HbA1c, urea and electrolytes, fasting lipid and fasting glucose levels, liver function tests, weight and blood pressure.

▶ Specific drugs require additional follow-up tests:
  ▷ serum prolactin levels if symptoms arise when using amisulpride, olanzapine, risperidone or zotepine
  ▷ annual full blood count for olanzapine, ziprasidone and aripiprazole
  ▷ measurement of creatine phosphokinase levels where symptoms of neuroleptic malignant syndrome arise
  ▷ annual thyroid function tests for quetiapine.

Method

Data collection

▶ An audit tool facilitated data collection. It was designed for easy recording of the name of antipsychotic used, date prescribed, and whether general and specific baseline and follow-up standards had been met.

▶ Data were collected from the medical notes and drug charts of patients.

Data analysis

The percentage of patients who had met each of the standards was calculated.

Resources required

People

One person can easily undertake the audit for the small numbers of patients on an in-patient unit. If carried out in the out-patient setting, where larger numbers of patients are likely, more data collectors would be helpful.

Time

It should be feasible to complete the audit within 4–5 hours, depending on the availability of case notes.

Results

- ▶ Overall, 78% of patients had had baseline blood tests.
- ▶ Performance was poor in relation to follow-up blood tests.

Recommendations

- ▶ Ward staff should flag up when tests are due, in ward rounds or meetings for the care programme approach.
- ▶ General practitioners should have an input into units to oversee the monitoring.
- ▶ Monitoring charts should be placed in an easily accessible area (e.g. clinic or drug sheet file).

Taylor, D., Paton, C. & Kerwin, R. (2007) *The Maudsley Prescribing Guidelines* (9th edition). Informa Healthcare.

82. Behavioural problems in adults with intellectual disabilities: medication management

Gemma Unwin and Shoumitro Deb

Setting

This audit is relevant to any setting where medication is prescribed to manage behavioural problems in adults with intellectual disabilities.

Background

Deb & Fraser (1994) estimated that 20–45% of people with intellectual disabilities take psychotropic medications, of whom 14–30% take them to control a behavioural problem such as aggression or self-injurious behaviour. Clarke *et al* (1990) reported that 36% of people with intellectual disabilities in residential settings are prescribed psychotropic medications in the absence of a diagnosed psychiatric illness. The aim of the audit was to investigate the practice and subsequent documentation of the use of medication in this context, as controversy surrounds it and there is a paucity of evidence of its effectiveness.

Standards

The standards were derived from a national guideline document (Deb *et al*, 2006):

▶ The prescriber needs to ensure that an assessment has been conducted and recorded before treatment is begun.

▶ The prescriber is responsible for assessing the person's capacity to consent to treatment.

▶ The prescriber should provide the person and/or carers with a written treatment plan at the time of prescribing. The prescriber should also discuss with the person and/or carers the common and serious adverse events related to the treatment (where possible, the prescriber should provide accessible information in writing).

▶ The method and timing of the assessment of outcome should be set at the beginning of the treatment, along with a follow-up date of review. As far as possible, there should be an objective way to assess outcome (the use of standardised scales is recommended).

▶ As far as possible, only one medication should be used at a time, within the recommended range of doses set out in the *British National Formulary* (*BNF*) (Joint Formulary Committee, 2009).

Method

Data collection

Investigators identified a list of all patients who were prescribed medication for a behavioural problem within the past 3 years. This may require investigation into the case notes of each patient within a clinic to establish the reason for any prescriptions. Cases where medication had been prescribed primarily for a mental illness, epilepsy, substance misuse or brain injury were excluded. The relevant case notes were examined to assess adherence to the recommendations.

Data extraction was completed using an audit questionnaire (see http://www.ld-medication.bham.ac.uk/technical.shtml).

Data analysis

The data were analysed to provide a percentage for the adherence of all the case notes to each of the recommendations.

Resources required

People

It may be advisable for more than one person to collect the data, to facilitate a larger yield of included case notes. If the audit is to be undertaken by more than one person, it is suggested that the audit team meets to discuss the level of evidence that is accepted as showing that the audit standard was adhered to.

Time

It should take 30–60 minutes to extract the data from each set of case notes, although this may depend on the length and complexity of the notes.

Results

In this multi-centre audit, 154 sets of case notes were reviewed. Most of them documented some assessment of the behaviour, defined the target behaviour, considered the use of non-medication-based interventions and noted the review date. However, issues around consent to treatment and capacity were poorly documented, as was documenting that a written treatment plan and written information on adverse effects had been handed to the person and/or carer.

Recommendations

▶ Compliance with these audit standards should be recorded in the case notes – a comprehensive clinic letter that covers the audit recommendations can facilitate this (see Deb *et al*, 2006, p. 37).

▶ There should be effective communication between the prescriber and person with intellectual disabilities and/or their carer – a written treatment plan and accessible medication information can facilitate this (see Deb *et al*, 2006, p. 39, and accessible information available at http://www.ld-medication.bham.ac.uk).

Clarke, D., Kelley, S., Thinn, K., *et al* (1990) Psychotropic drugs and mental retardation: 1. Disabilities and the prescription of drugs for behaviour and for epilepsy in three residential settings. *Journal of Mental Deficiency Research*, **28**, 229–233.

Deb, S. & Fraser, W. (1994) The use of psychotropic medication in people with learning disability: towards rational prescribing. *Human Psychopharmacology*, **9**, 259–272.

Deb, S., Clarke, D. & Unwin, G. (2006) *Using Medication to Manage Behaviour Problems Among Adults With a Learning Disability: Quick Reference Guide*. University of Birmingham, Mencap and the Royal College of Psychiatrists. Available http://www.ld-medication.bham.ac.uk (accessed October 2010).

Joint Formulary Committee (2009) *British National Formulary* (58th edition). British Medical Association & Royal Pharmaceutical Society of Great Britain.

Acknowledgement

The above audit was fully detailed in a previous publication: Gemma L. Unwin & Shoumitro Deb, 'A multi-centre audit of the use of medication for the management of behavioural problems in adults with intellectual disabilities'. *British Journal of Learning Disabilities*, **36**, Copyright© 2007 Blackwell Publishing Ltd.

83. Benzodiazepines in old age psychiatry

Ziad Tayar

Setting

This audit is relevant to both organic and functional disorders, and to acute assessment, rehabilitation and long-stay settings.

Background

Guidelines recommend the use of benzodiazepines for the short-term relief of severe anxiety or insomnia. However, clinical experience suggests that in old age psychiatry these drugs may be being prescribed for other indications.

Standards

The standards were taken from the *British National Formulary*, sections 4.1.1 and 4.1.2 (Joint Formulary Committee, 2009).

▶ Hypnotics should be for short-term use only (2–4 weeks).

▶ Anxiolytics should be prescribed for the relief of severe anxiety, at the lowest possible dose for the shortest possible time (2–4 weeks).

▶ Benzodiazepines can also be used as antimanic agents, in the initial stages of treatment, until mood stabilisers/antimanic drugs achieve their full effect.

▶ In panic disorders resistant to antidepressant therapy, a benzodiazepine (lorazepam or clonazepam, both of which are unlicensed) may be used. Alternatively, benzodiazepines may be used as short-term adjunctive therapy at the start of antidepressant treatment.

▶ Only one benzodiazepine should be used at a time.

The aim is to follow the prescribing guidelines and to have the reasons for benzodiazepine treatment documented in all instances.

Method

Data collection

A purpose-designed data-collection form was used, mainly in 'tick list' format, to make it easier and quicker to fill in. The following benzodiazepines were included on the data-collection form: lorazepam, oxazepam, zopiclone, alprazolam, diazepam, zaleplon, nitrazepam, chlordiazepoxide, lormetazepam, temazepam, zolpidem, flurazepam, clobazam, clorazepate and loprazolam.

Fifty randomly selected patients were included in the audit. This was done by selecting every third patient from a list of admissions to both acute and long-stay old age psychiatry wards. Information was collected jointly from the medication cards and the patients' medical notes.

Data analysis

The following information was collected:

▶ the proportion of patients prescribed benzodiazepines, broken down by gender

▶ the duration of use (less than or more than 4 weeks) and the type of use (as required or regular)

- the number of benzodiazepines prescribed per patient
- the indications for prescribing benzodiazepines.

Resources required

People

This audit is particularly suitable for multidisciplinary involvement, for example the pharmacist and a psychiatric trainee.

Time

For 50 cases, it is estimated that the data collection will take approximately 10 hours to complete. If electronic notes or prescribing records are available this will reduce the time required.

Results

- Overall, 72% of patients were prescribed one benzodiazepine.
- Overall, 28% had been prescribed more than one benzodiazepine concurrently.
- A benzodiazepine was prescribed to patients for more than 4 weeks on 100% of the long-stay wards and 65% of acute wards.
- Lorazepam was the most commonly used benzodiazepine (50% of all prescriptions).
- The most common reason for prescribing benzodiazepines was anxiety and agitation (64% of cases).
- In the case notes there was poor documentation of the reasons for prescribing benzodiazepines and of any discussions with patients.
- All prescriptions were within the *BNF* dose range, including regular and 'as required' use.

Recommendations

- The need to continue on benzodiazepine treatment should be reviewed regularly, especially for patients on long-stay wards.
- A process for improved documentation of the reasons for prescribing and of discussions with patients should be considered.

Joint Formulary Committee (2009) *British National Formulary* (58th edition). British Medical Association & Royal Pharmaceutical Society of Great Britain.

84. Covert administration of medication

Neel Halder, Nasim Chaudhry, Stewart Durairaj and Yaseem Aslam

Setting

This audit can be applied to in-patients or out-patients. It is relevant to all specialties of psychiatry, but especially psychiatry of old age and intellectual disability, where patients are more likely to lack capacity.

Background

Covert medication involves the administration of any pharmacological agent in a disguised form (usually hidden in food or drink). This leads to the patient ingesting an agent without having given explicit consent. The administration of covert medication is an ethically sensitive but pervasive practice in many healthcare settings. It has been a widely held misconception among healthcare professionals that the law allows for this practice, provided that it is in the patient's best interests. This confusion, with lack of clarity and guidance, has led to practices that could be deemed as indefensible in a court setting.

Standards

Standards were obtained from various sources including: the Royal College of Psychiatrists' statement on the covert administration of medicines (2004); the Mental Welfare Commission for Scotland's document *Covert Administration: Legal and Practical Guidance* (2006); the Mental Capacity Act 2005 (Department of Constitutional Affairs, 2007); and the Nursing and Midwifery Council's *Position Statement on Covert Administration of Medicines* (2001).

The following were the agreed audit standards:

▶ There should be a covert medications policy.
▶ The treatment must be necessary and in the best interest of the patient.
▶ For patients who are given medications covertly, there should be a written care plan that has been subject to consultation with the multidisciplinary team.
▶ The care plan and decision for covert use should be reviewed weekly initially, unless there is good justification for not doing this.
▶ There should be a written record of assessment of capacity, and reasons for presumed incapacity should be clearly documented.
▶ Covert administration should be seen as the least restrictive option.

The target was that all of the above standards were met.

Method

Data collection

▶ A list of all adults with intellectual disability with mental health needs should be kept by the local community intellectual disability team, and be obtainable electronically. If numbers are large, a random selection of carers can be used. For in-patient units, carers of all in-patients can be contacted.
▶ Carers and nursing staff were asked to fill in a questionnaire asking about compliance with the above standards. The questionnaire comprised specific yes/no questions but had some boxes for the entry of free text at the end.

Data analysis

The numbers of patients who were given medication covertly was calculated. The percentage of patients for whom the above standards were met was calculated.

Resources required

People

It is suggested that this audit is undertaken by at least three people, owing to the potentially large amount of information to collect and chase up. It is suitable for multidisciplinary involvement.

Time

Each questionnaire takes approximately 5 minutes to fill in. It is envisaged the majority of the time will be spent chasing up non-responders. For an average of 60 patients, at least 4–6 weeks should be allowed for most forms to be returned.

Results

Few carers stated they were using medicines covertly. In the vast majority of those cases where covert medications had been used, there was no policy in place, nor was there a documented capacity assessment. Often members of the multidisciplinary team were not consulted. Many areas for improvement were identified.

Recommendations

▶ The findings of the audit should be disseminated among carers of audited patient groups.
▶ Education of carers in routine clinical practice should be encouraged.
▶ A local policy on covert administration of medication should be developed.

Department of Constitutional Affairs (2007) *Code of Practice: Mental Capacity Act 2005*. The Stationery Office.

Mental Welfare Commission for Scotland (2006) *Covert Administration: Legal and Practical Guidance*. Mental Welfare Commission for Scotland. Available at http://www.mwcscot.org.uk/web/FILES/Publications/covertmedication.pdf (accessed October 2010).

Nursing & Midwifery Council (2001) *UKCC Position Statement on Covert Administration of Medicines*. Nursing and Midwifery Council. Available at http://www.nmc-uk.org/Publications-/Circulars/Nursing-circulars (accessed October 2010).

Royal College of Psychiatrists (2004) Statement on covert administration of medicines. *Psychiatric Bulletin*, **28**, 385–386. Available at http://pb.rcpsych.org/cgi/content/full/28/10/385 (accessed October 2010).

85. Depot antipsychotics: side-effects

Sheena Mitchell and Clare Oakley

Setting

This audit is relevant to any psychiatrist who prescribes depot antipsychotics; in general adult and forensic services it will apply to a large number of patients. It can apply to in-patients as well as out-patients.

Background

The Prescribing Observatory for Mental Health (POMH-UK) runs national audit-based quality improvement programmes open to all specialist mental health services in the UK. The aim is to help mental health services to improve prescribing practice in discrete areas. This audit addresses the quality of assessment of side-effects in patients prescribed depot or long-acting injections of antipsychotics. The decision was taken to limit the audit sample to patients prescribed depot antipsychotic medication because such patients have regular contact with health professionals when they receive their injection, which should provide an opportunity for routine monitoring of side-effects.

Standards

The National Institute for Health and Clinical Excellence (NICE) (2009) provides the following standards:

▶ Antipsychotic side-effects should be monitored routinely and regularly.
▶ People receiving depot preparations should be maintained under regular clinical review, particularly in relation to the risks and benefits of the medication.

From the above targets POMH derived a minimum standard of review of side-effects once a year for all patients prescribed depot or long-acting injection antipsychotics. It was expected that this would be achieved for 100% of patients.

Method

Data collection

All patients prescribed depot or long-acting injection antipsychotics were identified using prescribing data from the pharmacy department. The medical records of the identified patients were examined to determine compliance with the standard of documented annual review of side-effects.

Data analysis

▶ Basic demographic data were collected to aid understanding of the audit data, for example:
  ▷ age
  ▷ gender
  ▷ responsible clinician
  ▷ diagnosis
  ▷ type and dose of depot or long-acting injection.

▶ In addition to determining whether there was documentation relating to any side-effects it was useful specifically to consider whether there was a record of:
  ▷ weight gain
  ▷ movement disorders
  ▷ sexual side-effects
  ▷ menstrual abnormalities.
▶ If patients were experiencing side-effects, it should be noted whether appropriate action was taken (e.g. blood test for prolactin level, consideration of medication for extrapyramidal side-effects).
▶ The percentage of patients with an enquiry relating to side-effects was calculated.

Resources required

People
Depending on the size of the sample, this audit can be undertaken by one person if electronic medical records are used in the trust. If paper notes have to be examined, it is likely to require two people. This audit is particularly suitable for multidisciplinary involvement, for example a pharmacist or community psychiatric nurse.

Time
For the data collection of the 120 patients in this audit, it took approximately 6 hours, as medical records were electronic. It is likely to take longer with paper-based notes.

Results
▶ National results showed that there was no documentation of side-effects in the past year for 35% of patients taking depot medication.
▶ Locally there was no documentation for 28% of patients.
▶ A third of patients had a documented movement disorder.
▶ Documented assessment of sexual side-effects and menstrual irregularities was found to be particularly uncommon.
▶ No patients had a documented physical examination specifically to assess side-effects.

Recommendations
▶ A section specifically relating to sexual side-effects should be added to the annual physical health check form.
▶ Annual physical health checks for out-patients should be initiated by community psychiatric nurses, including measurement of weight.
▶ The audit should be extended to consider all patients prescribed antipsychotics, not just those on depots and long-acting injections.

National Institute for Health and Clinical Excellence (2009) *Schizophrenia: Core Interventions in the Treatment and Management of Schizophrenia in Primary and Secondary Care* (CG82). NICE. Available at http://guidance.nice.org.uk/CG82 (accessed October 2010).

86. Diazepam as rescue medication in epilepsy

Asit B. Biswas, Tracy Hobbs, Anthony Bailey, Dave Ball, Gordon Walker,
Sabyasachi Bhaumik and Agnes Hauck

Setting

This audit is particularly relevant where family carers and professional care staff look after people with intellectual disability and epilepsy, at home, in day care, in respite care and in the community.

Background

Epileptic seizures occur in a third of patients with severe intellectual disability. Previously it was common practice to attempt to treat status epilepticus with diazepam per rectum, but this can be difficult without appropriate training for carers and be embarrassing and undignified for the patient.

Standards

No national standards were available at the time. Seven good-practice standards were set, after discussion with professionals and carers:

▶ Adequate information is provided to carers regarding
  ▷ identification of a prolonged seizure
  ▷ identification of repeated seizures
  ▷ recognition of seizure type
  ▷ assessment of level of consciousness.
▶ The rationale for use of diazepam per rectum is explained.
▶ Clear written guidelines are provided for the timely administration of per rectum diazepam in relation to the first and second doses.
▶ Adequate training is given on the administration and dose of per rectum diazepam.
▶ Adequate information is provided on recognising the following complications after prolonged or repeated seizures:
  ▷ convulsive status epilepticus
  ▷ non-convulsive status epilepticus
  ▷ cyanosis
  ▷ aspiration and breathing difficulties
  ▷ in addition, adequate explanation is given on monitoring pulse, temperature and breathing after prolonged or repeated seizures.
▶ Adequate information is provided on when to call 999 for an ambulance.
▶ From the guidelines provided and training received, does the carer feel confident
  ▷ in identifying when per rectum diazepam is indicated
  ▷ with the procedure
  ▷ in identifying any complications that may result from administration of this drug
  ▷ in timing the decision to seek emergency help (dial 999).

Method

Data collection

All patients with intellectual disability and epilepsy identified as receiving or being prescribed diazepam per rectum for prolonged and/or repeated seizures over the audit period were included. Questionnaires were sent out to home carers, the day centre key worker or other staff and staff of respite care homes. An explanatory letter was provided explaining the aims and scope of the audit.

Data analysis

The percentage of the sample meeting each standard was calculated.

Resources required

People

This audit was led by a consultant intellectual disability psychiatrist and four community intellectual disability nurses incorporated it into their routine work as part of good clinical governance.

Time

It is estimated that each queationnaire takes 15–30 minutes to complete.

Results

▶ Overall, 86% reported that adequate information was provided to aid identification of a prolonged seizure, repetitive seizures and the type of seizure, and adequate training provided to administer diazepam per rectum.

▶ Over half (54%) received adequate information regarding assessment of the level of consciousness.

▶ The majority (91%) were provided with an explanation of the rationale for use of diazepam.

▶ Over two-thirds received information about complications (except non-convulsive status epilepticus) and when to call an ambulance.

▶ Overall, 64% found administration of diazepam per rectum convenient, 46% believed it to be comfortable for the patient, 41% thought it to be effective and 55% said that the patient needed to be moved to a more private area before diazepam could be administered.

▶ Under half (41%) preferred a buccal or intranasal route of administering rescue medication.

Recommendations

▶ Clearly presented information should be provided to carers and staff, in order to aid the identification of seizures and assessment of the level of consciousness.

▶ Clearly written guidelines for each individual patient should be provided for the timely administration of the two doses of diazepam per rectum. Easily accessible training opportunities should be made available to epilepsy specialist nurses and community intellectual disability nurses on the administration (and dose) of diazepam per rectum.

▶ Alternative forms of medication (e.g. buccal/intranasal midazolam) should be identified.

87. Electroconvulsive therapy: facilities

Sobia Khan

Setting

This audit is of particular relevance to old age and general adult psychiatric services.

Background

Despite the publication by the Royal College of Psychiatrists (1995) of detailed standards for the provision of electroconvulsive therapy (ECT), a three-cycle audit (Duffett & Lelliott, 1998) highlighted deficiencies in equipment and training and supervision of junior psychiatrists.

Standards

The standards were obtained from the ECT Accreditation Service (Royal College of Psychiatrists, 2003):

- ▶ The ECT clinic should comprise a minimum of three rooms, be clean, comfortable, welcoming, of adequate size, easily accessible and have toilet facilities.
- ▶ The clinic should have a small fridge and secure drug storage cupboard.
- ▶ Protocols for anaphylaxis, malignant hypertension and cardiac arrest should be displayed.
- ▶ Physical assessment of patients before ECT should include as a minimum:
  - ▷ a recent complete medical history and full examination
  - ▷ details of any previous anaesthetics or operations
  - ▷ a full list of the patient's prescribed drugs and allergies.
- ▶ The equipment should include:
  - ▷ recording ECT machine and patient trolleys
  - ▷ oxygen intermittent positive pressure ventilation, with one face mask per patient
  - ▷ cardiac arrest tray, suction machine and intravenous infusion sets
  - ▷ pulse oximeter, capnograph, electrocardiographic monitor, defibrillator, laryngoscope and blood glucose monitor.
- ▶ Drugs available in the clinic should include:
  - ▷ anaesthetic induction agent (propofol, thiopentone)
  - ▷ muscle relaxant (suxamethonium)
  - ▷ atropine, glycopyrolate, midazolam, naltrexone and dantrolene.
- ▶ Staff in clinic areas should consist of:
  - ▷ a senior nurse with special responsibility for ECT
  - ▷ a trained nurse in each of the treatment rooms and the recovery area
  - ▷ an untrained staff member in the waiting area
  - ▷ one person competent in cardiopulmonary resuscitation and one advanced life support provider
  - ▷ a named consultant psychiatrist (ECT lead) with a dedicated ECT session
  - ▷ a named lead clinician for anaesthesia for ECT and a trained assistant present during treatment

> ▷ doctors administering ECT, trained in the theoretical basis of ECT and familiar with local policy and procedure and clinic layout, and directly supervised at least three times before they perform unsupervised administration.
> ► Policies and procedures should be available with guidance on what settings to use to induce seizures, what to do in the absence of a seizure and when to terminate a prolonged seizure.

Method

Data collection

► Facilities, equipment, practice, personnel and training were systemically evaluated against ECTAS standards in all ECT clinics in the trust.
► At all clinics, treatment sessions were observed to determine whether the standards for assessment and practice were met.
► A small survey of doctors administering ECT was carried out to determine whether they had received adequate training and supervision.

Data analysis

Clinics were rated using a schedule of the ECTAS standards. Some standards (e.g. presence of equipment) were rated as present or absent, while others (e.g. rooms, personnel and training) were rated as poor, average or good.

Resources required

People

Up to three people may be needed to audit a large trust.

Time

To observe treatment sessions and carry out a survey of the doctors administering ECT a total of 4 weeks was required.

Results

The audit showed that all clinics met the required standards for ECT facilities and standards for anaesthetic staff. The audit identified some areas of concern:
► lack of emergency drugs
► some items of non-functional equipment
► staffing problems and poor patient identification processes, including lack of allocated session time for consultants to administer and supervise ECT.

Recommendations

► Equipment and written protocols should be standardised.
► A meeting should be held with management to consider resources in relation to equipment and staffing.

Duffett, R. & Lelliott, P. (1998) Auditing electroconvulsive therapy, the third cycle. *British Journal of Psychiatry*, 172, 401–405.
Royal College of Psychiatrists (1995) *The ECT Handbook: The 2nd Report of the Royal College of Psychiatrists' Special Committee on ECT*. RCPsych.
Royal College of Psychiatrists (2003) *ECT Accreditation Service: Standards for the Administration of ECT*. RCPsych (www.rcpsych.ac.uk/PDF/ECTAS%20Standards%202009.pdf).

88. Electroconvulsive therapy: indications

Isu Katuwawela

Setting

This audit is relevant to all psychiatric specialties but particularly older-adult services, where electroconvulsive therapy (ECT) may be more widely used.

Background

Although ECT is an effective treatment, it has the potential for serious adverse effects. The National Institute for Health and Clinical Excellence (NICE) (2003) has produced guidance relating specifically to the indications for ECT, the risks and benefits of treatment, consent, cessation of treatment and repeat courses of ECT.

Standards

The audit standards were taken from the NICE guidance (NICE, 2003):

▶ ECT should be used only to achieve rapid and short-term improvement of severe symptoms after an adequate trial of other treatment options has proven ineffective and/or when the condition is considered to be potentially life-threatening, in individuals with severe depressive illness, catatonia or a prolonged/severe manic episode.

▶ The decision whether ECT is clinically indicated should be based on assessment of the risks and potential benefits to the individual. These include anaesthetic risks, comorbidities, anticipated adverse events (especially cognitive impairment) and the risks of not having treatment.

▶ Valid consent should be obtained in all cases.

▶ Clinical status should be assessed following each ECT session. Treatment should be stopped when a response has been achieved, or sooner if there is evidence of adverse effects. Cognitive function should be monitored on an ongoing basis, and as a minimum at the end of each course of treatment.

▶ A repeat course of ECT should be considered only for individuals who have severe depressive illness, catatonia or mania and who have previously responded well to ECT. During an acute episode, if the patient has not previously responded, a repeat trial of ECT should be undertaken only after all other options have been considered and following discussion of the risks and benefits.

▶ ECT is not recommended as a maintenance therapy in depressive illness.

▶ ECT is not recommended for the general management of schizophrenia.

Method

Data collection

Information collected was obtained from medical notes and included:

▶ diagnosis
▶ reason for ECT
▶ risks and benefits of ECT

▶ consent for ECT
▶ cessation of ECT
▶ repeat courses of ECT
▶ use of ECT as maintenance therapy for depression or management of schizophrenia.

Data analysis
The proportion of cases meeting the required standards was calculated.

Resources required
People
It is possible for this audit to be conducted by one person.

Time
A total of seven patients received ECT during the audited period, and for these the data collection took around 4 hours.

Results
▶ Seven patients underwent ECT. The registration form in the ECT booklet was present in all seven sets of case records audited. ECT was administered because all other treatment options had proved ineffective in all cases.
▶ All patients who underwent ECT had a severe depressive illness. Six patients had their medical history and reason for ECT documented.
▶ In all cases, the benefits of ECT were discussed and documented in the clinical notes. There had been an improvement in the recording of the clinical status after each session and monitoring of cognitive function by the end of each course of treatment since an earlier audit.
▶ Four of the seven patients stopped ECT before the planned end of the treatment because a clinical response had been achieved. Only one patient out of seven received a repeat course of ECT.
▶ In one of seven patients, ECT was used as maintenance therapy for severe depressive illness. No patients received maintenance ECT for schizophrenia.

Recommendations
▶ The trust's ECT guidance policy should be revised to reflect available NICE guidance, to improve adherence.

National Institute for Health and Clinical Excellence (2003) *Guidance on the Use of Electroconvulsive Therapy* (TA59). NICE. Available at http://www.nice.org.uk/nicemedia/live/11494/32597/32597.pdf (accessed October 2010).

Acknowledgements
The original audit was conducted by S. Daniel and I. Braide and collated by the Clinical Audit Department, Birmingham and Solihull Mental Health NHS Foundation Trust.

89. Hypnotics

Josie Jenkinson

Setting

This audit is relevant to any in-patient setting where a significant proportion of patients may be prescribed hypnotics for the treatment of insomnia.

Background

The National Institute for Health and Clinical Excellence (NICE) (2004) has made several recommendations regarding the use of hypnotics for the treatment of insomnia. Insomnia is a symptom often experienced by those suffering from mental illness, and so hypnotics are frequently prescribed within psychiatric in-patient settings.

Standards

Standards were obtained from the audit criteria recommended by the National Institute for Health and Clinical Excellence (2004). These are as follows:

▶ Non-pharmacological measures are to be considered before the prescription of drug therapy for insomnia.
▶ When used, hypnotic drug therapy should be used for the shortest time necessary, and in strict accordance with the licensed indications.
▶ When hypnotic therapy is prescribed, the drug with the lowest purchase cost should be chosen. (The information on purchasing costs was obtained from the chief pharmacist.)
▶ Patients should not be switched from one drug to another.

The target was that these standards should be met for all in-patients prescribed hypnotics for insomnia.

Method

Data collection

Data were collected by examining the medical notes and prescription charts of all in-patients within the trust for evidence of the four standards. This was done as a snapshot audit over a pre-specified 2-week period.

Data analysis

The percentage of patients being prescribed hypnotics for insomnia for whom each of the following standards was met was calculated:

▶ documentation of the consideration of non-pharmacological measures
▶ hypnotic prescription not lasting for longer than 4 weeks
▶ drug with the lowest purchase cost used
▶ no switch from one drug to another.

The prescribing practices of different units was depicted through the use of pie charts and bar graphs.

Resources required

People

This audit would need to be completed by three or four people, depending on the size of the trust.

Time

For a trust with 250 in-patients, with approximately half of these being prescribed night sedation, it is estimated that data collection would take 20 hours.

Results

▶ Documentation of discussions relating to non-pharmacological measures, such as sleep hygiene, was almost universally absent.

▶ Compliance with length of prescription of hypnotics was good.

▶ Only one patient was switched from one hypnotic to another.

▶ The vast majority of patients were prescribed zopiclone, whereas the drug with the lowest purchase cost was diazepam.

Recommendations

▶ Local guidelines on the use of hypnotics should be developed, as the administration of controlled drugs adds significantly to the costs of using benzodiazepines.

▶ A sleep hygiene poster should be displayed on all in-patient wards and a leaflet on the subject should be made available.

▶ A checklist for review of hypnotics and symptoms of insomnia should be developed for use on ward rounds.

▶ A memorandum should be sent to all in-patient staff, reminding them of the importance of both non-pharmacological methods of managing insomnia and of good practice in prescribing.

▶ In addition, it was noted that psychiatric in-patient groups have specific needs and safety issues as regards hypnotic prescription (e.g. dependency issues, overdosing), which are not addressed by the NICE guidance.

National Institute for Health and Clinical Excellence (2004) *Guidance on the Use of Zaleplon, Zolpidem and Zopiclone for the Short-Term Management of Insomnia* (TA77). NICE. Available at http://www.nice.org.uk/nicemedia/pdf/TA077fullguidance.pdf (accessed October 2010).

90. Lithium: monitoring

Neil Masson

Setting

This audit is relevant to all psychiatrists prescribing lithium to out-patients.

Background

Lithium has an important place in the management of affective disorders but regular monitoring of blood and physical health is important to ensure its safe use. This monitoring is often done in a 'shared care' approach between the patient's psychiatrist and general practitioner. One downside of this is the potential for a breakdown in the effective monitoring of therapy.

Standards

The standards were obtained from a guideline on bipolar disorder produced by the National Institute for Health and Clinical Excellence (NICE) (2006). The relevant parts of this guideline include the following:

▶ the lithium level should be checked every 3 months
▶ urea and electrolytes and thyroid function should be checked every 6 months
▶ urea and electrolytes should be checked more often than every 6 months if the patient is taking angiotensin-converting enzyme (ACE) inhibitors, diuretics or non-steroidal anti-inflammatory drugs (NSAIDs)
▶ glucose and blood pressure should be checked annually
▶ lipids should be checked annually for patients aged over 40 years.

Method

Data collection

The computerised patient record system in a local general practice was used to identify all patients who were prescribed lithium from this practice and from sister practices. This system was used to collect data on:

▶ patient age
▶ diagnosis
▶ drug history
▶ date and results for:
  ▷ blood pressure
  ▷ lithium level
  ▷ thyroid function tests
  ▷ urea and electrolytes
  ▷ glucose
  ▷ lipids.

Data analysis

The main outcome measure was the percentage of patients taking lithium who had had adequate monitoring of blood pressure, lithium level, thyroid function, urea and electrolytes, glucose and lipids.

Resources required

People

Only one person is required to conduct this audit, but if that person is unfamiliar with the computerised system the practice uses, help from a staff member at the practice may be needed.

Time

This will depend on the size of the practice, but it is estimated that all information could be obtained from the practice computer system in around 8 hours.

Results

- ► The percentage of patients who had adequate monitoring of urea and electrolytes, thyroid function and lithium level was good.
- ► The percentage of patients who had adequate monitoring of glucose and blood pressure was low.
- ► Those patients who were on specified medications who were required to have more frequent monitoring of urea and electrolytes did not.
- ► The percentage of those over 40 who had annual lipid monitoring was also low.
- ► After implementing the steps below the situation had improved dramatically at a re-audit.

Recommendations

- ► The results of the audit were presented to general practitioners as part of a practice meeting, along with the salient features of the NICE guideline.
- ► Those patients who did not have adequate monitoring were 'tagged' by the practice computer system to ensure the necessary monitoring was done next time they visited for blood tests.

National Institute for Health and Clinical Excellence (2006) *Bipolar Disorder: The Management of Bipolar Disorder in Adults, Children and Adolescents, in Primary and Secondary Care* (CG38). NICE. Available at http://guidance.nice.org.uk/CG38 (accessed October 2010).

91. Medicines reconciliation

Rohit Bhardwaj

Setting

This audit is suited to investigating medication errors at the point of patient transfer between a variety of care settings.

Background

Medication errors are recognised as a common cause of avoidable morbidity and mortality (Dean-Franklin *et al*, 2005). Approximately 20% of clinical negligence claims on the part of hospitalised patients are due to medication errors (Audit Commission, 2001). The National Patient Safety Agency (NPSA) (2007), in conjunction with the National Institute for Health and Clinical Excellence (NICE), has defined medicines reconciliation as:

▶ collecting information on medication history (before admission) using the most recent and accurate sources to create a full and current list of medicines
▶ checking or verifying this list against the current hospital prescription chart
▶ ensuring any discrepancies are accounted for and actioned appropriately
▶ communicating any changes, omissions or discrepancies.

Standards

The NPSA (2007) makes the following recommendations:

▶ All healthcare organisations that admit adult in-patients should make sure that they have policies in place for medicines reconciliation on admission.
▶ In addition to specifying standardised systems for collecting and documenting information about current medications, policies for medicines reconciliation on admission should ensure that:
  ▷ pharmacists are involved as soon as possible after admission
  ▷ the responsibilities of pharmacists and other staff in the medicines reconciliation process are clearly defined
  ▷ strategies are incorporated to obtain information about medications for people with communication difficulties.

Method

Data collection

To assess whether an appropriate policy on medicines reconciliation was present, data were collected to answer the following questions:

▶ Does the organisation have an approved or draft policy?
▶ Which staff roles have responsibility for medicines reconciliation?
▶ Does the policy specify the time frame for reconciliation, which sources of information are required and where to document them?
▶ Has an earlier medicines reconciliation audit taken place?

To assess the quality of medicines reconciliation, data should be collected on a questionnaire/audit tool for a minimum of five consecutive in-patient admissions. The audit should be completed after the patient has been admitted for at least 7 days. The following data should be collected:

▶ documented details of medicines before admission (prescribed and non-prescribed), and adherence to these

▶ evidence of a team discussion regarding sources checked, discrepancies identified, and whether these are documented

▶ whether a member of the medicines management team has been involved and the timescale of this involvement.

Data analysis

Data can be analysed at organisational or team level. The Prescribing Observatory for Mental Health led the original audit, which allowed the data to be analysed on a national level. The percentages meeting the standards were calculated.

Resources required

People

For the assessment of the presence of an appropriate policy, the audit can be undertaken by one professional with a good knowledge of the organisational systems for managing medicines. Data for the in-patient audit can be collected by one professional with clinical expertise, for each clinical team.

Time

It is estimated that data collection for five in-patients would take anywhere between 2 and 5 hours.

Results

In relation to organisational policy:

▶ Approaching half (44%) of organisations did not have an approved policy for medicines reconciliation.

▶ For organisations that had a policy, the majority stated who was responsible for medicines reconciliation, the time frame in which it should take place and where the details should be recorded.

In relation to the in-patient audit:

▶ Discrepancies in the medication regimen were identified in 25% of the total national sample for whom two or more sources of information had been checked.

▶ Of the specific discrepancies reported, only a small proportion was clearly clinically significant.

Recommendations

The Prescribing Observatory for Mental Health is developing a patient-led intervention that highlights the importance of telling the doctor about all medicines that are currently being taken. Engagement by trusts/health boards in this process could improve awareness and lead to an improvement in attaining the standards.

Audit Commission (2001) *A Spoonful of Sugar – Medicines Management in NHS Hospitals*. Audit Commission.

Dean-Franklin, B., Vincent, C., Schachter, M., *et al* (2005) The incidence of prescribing errors in hospital inpatients: an overview of the research methods. *Drug Safety*, **28**, 891–900.

National Patient Safety Agency (2007) NICE/NPSA issues its first patient safety solution guidance to improve medicines reconciliation at hospital admission. At http://www.npsa.nhs.uk/corporate/news/guidance-to-improve-medicines-reconciliation (accessed October 2010).

92. Mood stabilisers: monitoring

Hannah Roberts and Debasish Das Purkayastha

Setting

This audit relates to all services where patients are treated for bipolar affective disorder or otherwise prescribed mood stabilisers. It relates to both in- and out-patients.

Background

The mood-stabilising drugs valproate and carbamazepine are widely prescribed within psychiatric services and each has its own list of potentially harmful adverse effects. (Lithium monitoring is considered in audit 90, p. 211.) As a result, there are important monitoring recommendations for both drugs. These include monitoring of the possible side-effects, as well as therapeutic drug monitoring, which aims to avoid the side-effects while ensuring therapeutic levels of the drug are achieved.

Standards

Standards for audit were obtained from the guideline on bipolar disorder produced by the National Institute for Health and Clinical Excellence (NICE) (2006):

▶ Patients prescribed valproate should have the following baseline assessments prior to initiation of treatment:
  ▷ liver function tests (LFTs)
  ▷ full blood count (FBC)
  ▷ weight and height.
▶ Patients prescribed valproate should have LFTs and FBC rechecked 6 months after initiation of treatment.
▶ Patients prescribed carbamazepine should have the following baseline assessments prior to initiation of treatment:
  ▷ LFTs
  ▷ FBC
  ▷ weight and height.
▶ Patients prescribed carbamazepine should have:
  ▷ LFTs, urea and electrolytes (U&Es) and FBC checked 6 months after initiation of treatment
  ▷ U&Es monitored every 6 months subsequent to this
  ▷ serum carbamazepine levels measured every 6 months.

It was expected that the standards would be met for 100% of patients.

Method

Data collection

A list of patients prescribed valproate or carbamazepine was created by examination of in-patient medication charts and out-patient records held in the pharmacy. The medical notes and online pathology results for each of these patients were then examined to determine which monitoring tests had been carried out over a previous defined period.

Data analysis

The percentage of patients who had undergone each test applicable to them was calculated and these percentages compared against the standards set above.

Resources required

People

Owing to the volume of notes to be read and the amount of data to collect and analyse, it is suggested that two people undertake this audit. It is appropriate that different disciplines are involved (e.g. a doctor and a pharmacist).

Time

For a service where a total of 30 patients are prescribed valproate or carbamazepine, the data collection and analysis should take about 10 hours.

Results

Compliance with the audit standards in a regional medium-secure unit was generally poor, with the exception of baseline tests for valproate.

Identified limitations of the audit included the audit period not being long enough to pick up some required tests, so some standards could not be measured, and notes were not checked for documented refusals of tests. Both these points should be considered in future audits.

Recommendations

▶ The audit results should be circulated to all clinical teams, together with a memorandum on the required monitoring tests for each of the two mood stabilisers.

▶ A form should be kept in the patient's notes when they are prescribed one of the two drugs with a table of the appropriate monitoring parameters to be completed as tests are done.

▶ A re-audit in 12 months should take account of the limitations of the present audit.

▶ Improved compliance with the standards set would improve patient safety, compliance with medication and clinician accountability.

National Institute for Health and Clinical Excellence (2006) *Bipolar Disorder: The Management of Bipolar Disorder in Adults, Children and Adolescents, in Primary and Secondary Care* (CG38). NICE. Available at http://guidance.nice.org.uk/CG38 (accessed October 2010).

93. Nurses' administration of medication

Mark Lovell and Laura Ramsay

Setting

This audit is relevant to an in-patient setting. It is designed to be completed in conjunction with the prescribing audits in relation to the *British National Formulary* (*BNF*) (audit 94, p. 219) and Mental Capacity Act (audit 95, p. 221).

Background

There are various pieces of legislation and various guidelines relating to the administration of medications (Royal Pharmaceutical Society, 2005; Nursing and Midwifery Council, 2007). If these are not adhered to, the result may be unlawful or unsafe practice. It is important for in-patient units to check that they are being lawful and following best practice.

This audit can be broken down into parts that are deemed relevant to a service. The audit can be done on all medication, just psychiatric medication, regular prescribing or 'as required' prescribing, or simply focused on one particular group of medicines or one patient group. There are guidelines for administering medication on wards. In addition to these, there are additional regulatory requirements for controlled drugs. Medicines currently classified as controlled drugs are listed in the current Misuse of Drugs Regulations (Home Office, 2009) and the *British National Formulary* (Joint Formulary Committee, 2009).

Standards

From the guidelines produced by the Royal Pharmaceutical Society (2005) and the Nursing and Midwifery Council (2007), the following standards in relation to nurses' administration of general drugs were used:

▶ A record of administration should be made (e.g. time and date).
▶ The administering nurse should be identified (e.g. signature or initials).
▶ Medication that is not given owing to refusal, wastage or lack of availability should be recorded.
▶ A record should be made when the task of administering medicine is delegated.
▶ The signature of a student administering medicines must be countersigned by a supervisor.

With specific reference to nurses' administration of controlled drugs, the standard was that the following details should be recorded in the 'Controlled Drug Register':

▶ date on which the issue was made
▶ name of the patient
▶ the amount of drug issued
▶ the form in which the drug was issued
▶ the name/signature of the nurse or authorised person making the issue
▶ the name/signature of a witness (nurse, student nurse, doctor or pharmacist)
▶ the balance of the drug left in stock
▶ the amount of drug given and the amount wasted (if part of a vial is given to the patient).

Method

Data collection

Data were collected retrospectively for a period of 3 months for all patients in a particular setting (e.g. for a particular team or ward). The data collected related to the presence of documentation in the nursing notes, on medication charts and in the Controlled Drugs Register. Each separate administration was checked for adherence to the standards for the audit.

Data analysis

The data were compared with the standards to estimate rates of compliance.

Resources required

People

This audit has the potential to be very large (when done in conjunction with audits 94 and 95) if all of the standards are considered. It is prudent to focus the audit according to service need. Owing to the amount of data to collect and the subsequent analysis, this part of the audit should be carried out by two members of nursing staff.

Time

This could be a short audit, looking at a cross-section of in-patients, through to a large time-consuming project. At least 1 hour should be allowed per set of notes.

Results

The original audit covered all 'as required' administration of medication for an adult intellectual disability in-patient unit. It found that there were good rates of adherence to the Nursing and Midwifery Council and Royal Pharmaceutical Society guidelines for general administering. However, there were some concerns around the administration of controlled drugs for sleep; this was highlighted by the fact that administration times slipped back each night because the medications were prescribed for 24 hours and then were 're-set' to a logical time against the prescribed maximum dose per 24 hours.

Recommendations

▶ It was suggested that hypnotics be prescribed per night rather than per 24 hours, to improve patient care.
▶ Refresher training pertaining to legislation and the administration of medication was also recommended.

Home Office (2009) Controlled Drugs List (updated January 2009) (http://www.homeoffice.gov.uk/publications/drugs/drug-licences/controlled-drugs-list). Home Office.

Joint Formulary Committee (2009) *British National Formulary* (58th edition). British Medical Association & Royal Pharmaceutical Society of Great Britain.

Nursing and Midwifery Council (2007) *Standards for Medicines Management.* NMC. Available at http://www.nmc-uk.org/Documents/Standards/nmcStandardsForMedicinesManagementBooklet.pdf (accessed October 2010).

Royal Pharmaceutical Society (2005) *The Safe and Secure Handling of Medicines: A Team Approach.* A revision of the Duthie Report (1988) led by the Hospital Pharmacists' Group of the Royal Pharmaceutical Society. RPSGB. Available at http://www.rpsgb.com/pdfs/safsechandmeds.pdf (accessed October 2010).

94. Prescribing: *British National Formulary* limits

Mark Lovell and Laura Ramsay

Setting

This audit is appropriate for all psychiatric in-patient settings. It is designed to be carried out in conjunction with the Mental Capacity Act audit (audit 95, p. 221) and the audit of nursing administration of medication (audit 93, p. 217).

Background

Prescribing of medication is governed by various legislative acts and guidelines. Adherence to these is important and it may even be unlawful or unsafe if medications are prescribed outside certain parameters. This audit can be broken down into parts that are deemed relevant by a service. The audit can be done on all medication, be restricted to psychiatric medication, regular prescribing or 'as required' prescribing (p.r.n.). The *British National Formulary* (*BNF*) is produced twice each year and gives guidance on the licensed uses for medications and their maximum doses (Joint Formulary Committee, 2009).

Standards

The *BNF* limits should be adhered to for each prescription of the medication in question. Below are sample adult *BNF* limits for oral psychiatric medications (see each relevant chapter of the most recent issue of the *BNF* for current dosage limits or medications not featured below):

▶ Hypnotics
  ▷ nitrazepam, 10 mg
  ▷ temazepam, 40 mg
  ▷ zopiclone, 7.5 mg
▶ Anxiolytics
  ▷ diazepam, 30 mg
  ▷ lorazepam, 4 mg
▶ Antipsychotics
  ▷ chlorpromazine, 1 g
  ▷ haloperidol, 30 mg
  ▷ amisulpride, 1.2 g
  ▷ aripiprazole, 30 mg
  ▷ clozapine, 900 mg
  ▷ olanzapine, 20 mg
  ▷ quetiapine, 750 mg
  ▷ risperidone, 16 mg
▶ Antimanics
  ▷ valproic acid, 2 g
  ▷ carbamazepine, 1.6 g
▶ Antidepressants
  ▷ venlafaxine, 375 mg
  ▷ citalopram, 60 mg

▷ fluoxetine, 80 mg

▷ mirtazepine, 45 mg

Method

Data collection

Data were collected retrospectively for a period of 3 months for all patients in a setting (e.g. for a particular team or ward). Data could also be collected prospectively after an intervention (e.g. a training session for relevant staff on *BNF* limits and prescribing). The data collected relate to the presence or absence of documentation of adherence to the above standard (e.g. documentation in medication charts of a maximum dose). Each separate prescription should be checked for adherence to the standard for the audit. Notes should also be taken of any idiosyncratic prescribing (even if it technically complies with the standards) and of any difficulties in finding the data.

Data analysis

The data were used to generate a percentage compliance rate with the standard.

Resources required

People

This audit has the potential to be very large if all the separate audits are considered. It is prudent to focus the audit according to service need. Owing to the amount of data to collect and the subsequent analysis, this audit should be carried out by two people.

Time

This can be a short audit, looking at a cross-section of in-patients, through to an enormous time-consuming project. At least 1 hour should be allowed per set of notes.

Results

The original audit covered all 'as required' prescribing (psychiatric and non-psychiatric) for an adult intellectual disability in-patient unit and found that all *BNF* limits were adhered to.

Recommendations

▶ Suggestions were made for future audits, such as to examine only psychiatric 'as required' prescribing (to focus the audit) or to examine all 'regular' prescribing (to expand the audit).

▶ A wider range of prescribing legislation and guidelines could be considered in future audits.

Joint Formulary Committee (2009) *British National Formulary* (58th edition). British Medical Association & Royal Pharmaceutical Society of Great Britain.

95. Prescribing: Mental Capacity Act

Mark Lovell and Laura Ramsay

Setting

This audit is appropriate for all psychiatric in-patient settings in England and Wales (with patients over 16 years of age). It is designed to be carried out in conjunction with the audits of nurses' administration of medication (audit 93, p. 217) and of the *British National Formulary* limits (audit 94, p. 219).

Background

The Mental Capacity Act 2005 provides a framework for people over the age of 16 years who lack capacity to make decisions for themselves, or who have capacity and want to make advance decisions in preparation for a time when they may lack capacity in the future. It sets out who can make decisions, and when and how they should go about this.

Standards

A code of practice (Department for Constitutional Affairs, 2007) has been produced to offer guidance on the Mental Capacity Act 2005.

The standard procedure for assessing capacity involves determination of the following:

▶ Does the person have an impairment of, or a disturbance in the functioning of, their mind or brain?

If so:

▶ Does the person understand information about the decision to be made?
▶ Can they retain that information in their mind?
▶ Can they use or weigh that information as part of the decision-making process?
▶ Can they communicate their decision (by talking, using sign language or any other means)?

Professionals should carry out an assessment of a person's capacity to make particular decisions and record the findings. It is important to review capacity from time to time, as a person's decision-making capabilities can change. Capacity should always be reviewed when decisions need to be made (e.g. for new medications).

Decisions may be made in the best interests of the person who lacks capacity to make those decisions for themselves (in the absence of an advance decision to refuse treatment by the person while having capacity). A record should be kept of best interests decisions for each relevant decision. This record should include:

▶ how the best interests decision was reached
▶ what the reasons for reaching the decision were
▶ who was consulted
▶ what factors were taken into account.

It was expected that for all people who lack capacity:

▶ The standard capacity assessment is documented for all new prescriptions.

▶ Any 'best interests' decisions are documented as per the code of practice.

Method

Data collection

Data were collected retrospectively for a period of 3 months for all patients in a setting (e.g. for a particular team or ward). The data related to the presence or absence of documentation of adherence to the above standards (e.g. documentation of capacity and 'best interests' decisions).

Data analysis

The data were used to generate a percentage compliance rate with the standard.

Resources required

People

This audit has the potential to be very large if all of the additional audits are considered. It is prudent to focus the audit according to service need. Owing to the amount of data to collect and the subsequent analysis, this audit should be carried out by two people.

Time

This can be a short audit, looking at a cross-section of in-patients, through to an enormous time-consuming project. At least 1 hour should be allowed for each set of notes.

Results

The original audit covered all 'as required' prescribing (psychiatric and non-psychiatric) for an adult intellectual disability in-patient unit. It found that improvements should be made to the assessment of capacity and 'best interests' documentation for new prescriptions.

Recommendations

▶ Suggestions were made to improve the documentation around the Mental Capacity Act 2005 and new prescriptions.

▶ Some of the data were hard to find since the design of the section headings used in the clinical notes preceded the Mental Capacity Act 2005 and thus the location of the documentation was *ad hoc*. A recommendation was made to address this issue and to document the relevant information in a new section of the notes.

Department for Constitutional Affairs (2007) *Mental Capacity Act 2005 Code of Practice*. The Stationery Office.

96. Prescribing: p.r.n. medication

Madhusudan Deepak Thalitaya

Setting

This audit will be relevant to all in-patient psychiatric settings where a high proportion of patients are prescribed medication 'as required' (p.r.n.).

Background

Prescribing p.r.n. is a common but valuable facility. Nonetheless, it is open to misuse and may be unnecessary or inappropriate (Department of Health, 2000). The Department of Health in 2000 committed itself to reducing serious prescribing errors by 40% by 2005. Prescribing errors are a daily occurrence in mental health trusts. The prescribing of p.r.n. antipsychotics is a contributor to combined and high-dose antipsychotic medication.

Standards

There are no national published 'gold standard' guidelines for p.r.n. prescribing. Generic standards were therefore obtained from the local trust's medicine policy and based on good clinical practice and principles (these could be used as a template for other teams aiming to audit the use of p.r.n. medication). All p.r.n. prescriptions should:

▶ use generic names (albeit with some exceptions)
▶ have a specified route of administration
▶ have each administration route prescribed separately
▶ show the maximum dose allowed in 24 hours
▶ show the minimum interval required between doses
▶ indicate whether the same drug (or class of drug) is also prescribed regularly
▶ involve only one drug from any one therapeutic category of the *British National Formulary* (*BNF*) (Joint Formulary Committee, 2009)
▶ be within *BNF* limits, unless high-dose prescribing is consented to (and, where more than one route is prescribed, in total this should still be within *BNF* limits or cross-referenced)
▶ have a specified review date and/or be reviewed at least once per month
▶ be cancelled if not used for longer than 1 month
▶ be reviewed if used on a regular basis (daily, for longer than 72 hours)
▶ have clear indications for use
▶ be rewritten if there are any alterations in the prescription.

The target is that these standards are met for all patients.

Method

Data collection

Data were collected over a 3-month period covering all the in-patients. Medical case records and drug charts were reviewed retrospectively. All p.r.n. prescriptions were reviewed against the standards.

Data analysis

The total percentage of compliance with the above standards was analysed using spreadsheet software.

Resources required

People

It is recommended that medical staff are involved in the audit process as it improves their prescribing by increasing awareness.

Time

For a service with nearly 70 patients, it is estimated that the data collection would take 12 hours and another 4 hours for data analysis.

Results

- ▶ Although there was a high number of p.r.n. prescriptions, nearly a quarter of patients were not on any p.r.n. medications.
- ▶ More than half the p.r.n. medications were for physical conditions. The remainder included antipsychotics, benzodiazepines, hypnotics and anticholinergic medications.
- ▶ There were more errors with prescriptions for physical conditions than for mental conditions.
- ▶ The audit showed excellent compliance with the majority of the standards. There was scope for improvement in relation to the following standards:
  - ▷ each administration route being subject to separate prescription
  - ▷ specifying a minimum interval between doses
  - ▷ having a specified review date.

Recommendations

- ▶ There should be regular review of p.r.n. prescriptions.
- ▶ A minimum interval between doses should be highlighted on all p.r.n. prescription forms, and there should be an indication of whether the drug is used regularly.
- ▶ The trust induction process for doctors should include p.r.n. standards in the induction pack and there should be annual reminders of these standards.
- ▶ Pharmacists should be regularly involved in ward rounds and reviews.
- ▶ Hospitals should have p.r.n. guidelines printed and circulated.
- ▶ Regular auditing, especially by medical and pharmaceutical staff, would enhance awareness of p.r.n. prescribing practice.

Department of Health (2000) *An Organisation with a Memory: Report of an Expert Group on Learning from Adverse Events in the NHS*. DH. Available at http://www.dh.gov.uk/en/Publicationsandstatistics/Publications/PublicationsPolicyAndGuidance/DH_4065083 (accessed October 2010).

Joint Formulary Committee (2009) *British National Formulary* (58th edition). British Medical Association & Royal Pharmaceutical Society of Great Britain.

97. Prescription charts

Victoria Lukats

Setting

This audit was carried out across all acute psychiatric in-patient wards in a district general hospital. It has since been repeated in other local psychiatric units with acute admission wards.

Background

Patients admitted to psychiatric units are frequently prescribed medication during their admission. Individual National Health Service (NHS) organisations will have their own guidelines as to how the prescription charts are to be completed and these will be based on guidelines in the *British National Formulary* (*BNF*) (Joint Formulary Committee, 2009). Guidelines are usually printed on the front of in-patient prescription charts. An audit of in-patient prescription charts is often a popular audit for junior doctors to undertake, as it can be completed quickly. This audit has proved popular locally and has been subject to re-audit on a number of occasions.

Standards

Standards were obtained from the *BNF* and from the guidelines printed on the front of the local in-patient prescription charts. Of particular relevance were the following:

▶ Prescription charts should be written in ink, using capital letters.
▶ The patient's name, date of birth and hospital number should appear on the front of the chart.
▶ The allergy section should be completed (it is not satisfactory to leave this blank or to write 'not known').
▶ Prescriptions should be legible.
▶ Each prescription should be signed and dated by the prescribing doctor.
▶ Approved generic drug names should be used unless inappropriate (e.g. where different preparations do not have the same bioavailability).
▶ Administration times should be clearly marked.
▶ The dosage should be clearly marked for each prescription.
▶ When a drug is discontinued, the individual prescription should be clearly crossed through in ink, signed and dated.
▶ For 'as required' (p.r.n.) medication, the indication should be clearly recorded and a single administration route should be specified for each drug prescription box.

The target is that these standards are met for all in-patient prescription charts.

Method

Data collection

A data-collection sheet was drawn up to record adherence to the above standards for each prescription chart audited. The prescription charts for all in-patients on a given day were identified. Each prescription chart in turn was then examined to determine whether the above standards had been met.

Data analysis

▶ The percentage of in-patient prescription cards meeting all standards was calculated.

▶ The percentage of individual prescription cards meeting each individual standard was calculated.

▶ The percentage of individual drug prescriptions meeting each standard relating to prescriptions was calculated.

Resources required

People

This audit can be carried out by a single junior doctor or by two or three working together.

Time

The data collection on 50–60 prescription charts could be carried out in a single day.

Results

Generally, the prescription charts were completed to a good standard, although it was not infrequent to find that corrections had been prompted by the hospital pharmacist. Specific areas for improvement were completing the allergy box, using capitals and discontinuing prescriptions by crossing through, signing and dating.

Recommendations

▶ The results of the audit should be fed back to all doctors during weekly academic meetings.

▶ Brief training on prescription charts should be incorporated into the junior doctors' induction.

▶ Regular re-audit should be undertaken, in order to monitor standards and to encourage good practice.

Joint Formulary Committee (2009) *British National Formulary* (58th edition). British Medical Association & Royal Pharmaceutical Society of Great Britain.

98. Psychological therapies

Lauren Coates

Setting

This audit was carried out in the alcohol and drug service, but it would be equally relevant to any general adult psychiatry or older persons' out-patient or in-patient service.

Background

The various guidelines on psychological therapies produced by the National Institute for Health and Clinical Excellence (NICE) (listed below) make clear recommendations regarding the provision for a number of common psychiatric conditions.

Standards

The standards were obtained from NICE guidelines:

▶ At a minimum, all patients with mild depression, generalised anxiety disorder, panic disorder or anorexia nervosa should be offered psychological therapy as the first-line treatment.

▶ Patients with moderate or severe depression or schizophrenia should be offered psychological therapy as an adjunct to medication.

The target is that all patients will be offered psychological therapies, as appropriate for their diagnosis, as suggested by the NICE guidelines.

Method

Data collection

For the purposes of this audit a computerised records system was used to identify a sample of 50 consecutive patients receiving an initial assessment. The assessment forms on the system were examined to acquire the information listed below. It is also possible to collect information prospectively, with the relevant information recorded each time an assessment is done.

Information required from the initial assessment was as follows:

▶ Were any psychiatric and/or psychological problems identified?

▶ If so, were these problems past or current?

▶ What treatment, if any, was the patient offered and by whom?

▶ What treatment, if any, did the patient receive and from whom?

Data analysis

The percentages of patients with current psychiatric and/or psychological problems and with past problems were calculated (one patient could be present in both subsets). For each of these subsets, the percentages of those receiving or who had received psychological therapies in line with NICE guidelines were calculated.

Resources required

People

This audit can be undertaken by one person for a sample of around 50 patients, although this will depend on the records system in use (it will be more time-consuming if paper notes have to be located and searched through). Where a team undertakes initial assessments, each member could be involved and could collect information as they go along.

Time

Data collection took around 6 hours for the original audit. The actual time will depend very much on the type of records system in use, the sample size and the number of people working together.

Results

None of the patients currently suffering with depression, anxiety or psychosis was receiving a psychological therapy. Very few of those currently being treated for other conditions were receiving a psychological therapy and the same was found for those treated for psychiatric or psychological problems in the past. There was a high level of unmet need with regard to the therapies suggested by the NICE guidelines.

Recommendations

▶ Ideally, each service should have a psychologist who can offer psychological therapies to all appropriate patients.

▶ Where there are high levels of unmet need, audit results could be brought before a governance committee or similar.

▶ Training should be given to other members of the multidisciplinary team to enable them to undertake structured interventions.

▶ More robust referral pathways to other services offering psychological therapies should be established.

▶ Any continuing unmet need should be identified and recorded as part of a complete audit cycle.

National Institute for Health and Clinical Excellence (2004) *Anxiety: Management of Anxiety (Panic Disorder, with or without Agoraphobia, and Generalised Anxiety Disorder) in Adults in Primary, Secondary and Community Care* (CG22). NICE. Available at http://guidance.nice.org.uk/CG22 (accessed October 2010).

National Institute for Health and Clinical Excellence (2004) *Eating Disorders: Core Interventions in the Treatment and Management of Anorexia Nervosa, Bulimia Nervosa and Related Eating Disorders* (CG9). NICE. Available at http://www.nice.org.uk/CG9 (accessed October 2010).

National Institute for Health and Clinical Excellence (2004) *Self-Harm: The Short Term Physical and Psychological Management and Secondary Prevention of Self-Harm in Primary and Secondary Care* (CG16). NICE. Available at http://www.nice.org.uk/Guidance/CG16 (accessed October 2010).

National Institute for Health and Clinical Excellence (2006) *Bipolar Disorder: The Management of Bipolar Disorder in Adults, Children and Adolescents, in Primary and Secondary Care* (Clinical Guideline 38). NICE. Available at http://guidance.nice.org.uk/CG38 (accessed October 2010).

National Institute for Health and Clinical Excellence (2009) *Borderline Personality Disorder: Treatment and Management* (CG78). NICE. Available at http://www.nice.org.uk/CG78 (accessed October 2010).

National Institute for Health and Clinical Excellence (2009) *Depression in Adults (Update)* (CG90). NICE. Available at http://guidance.nice.org.uk/CG90 (accessed October 2010).

National Institute for Health and Clinical Excellence (2009) *Schizophrenia: Core Interventions in the Treatment and Management of Schizophrenia in Primary and Secondary Care* (CG82). NICE. Available at http://guidance.nice.org.uk/CG82 (accessed October 2010).

99. Psychotherapy re-referrals

Lisa Gardiner

Setting

This audit is relevant in psychotherapy services and considers re-referrals after the patient had received 20 sessions of psychodynamic psychotherapy.

Background

Psychodynamic psychotherapy is one of the more commonly offered talking treatments in the National Health Service (NHS). It is usually offered on a once-weekly basis, with sessions lasting 50 minutes. The duration of treatment can range from 10 sessions or fewer (for brief therapies) to 6 months or less (moderate-length therapies) or 1 year or more (longer-term treatment).

Organising and Delivering Psychological Therapies (Department of Health, 2004) remains the most relevant publication for psychotherapy service delivery in secondary care. It also gives some direction on measuring service delivery. Two of its recommended action points for specialised mental health services are:

▶ contribute to the debate about the best performance indicators for psychological therapies – waiting times for psychology and psychotherapy assessment are the most promising

▶ extend the use of outcome measures across all aspects of psychological therapy service provision.

These action points can be extrapolated to standards that might apply to those individuals who have already been through the cycle of: assessment, referral, waiting list, therapy (a 'dose' of 20 sessions) and re-referral after unsuccessful treatment. These individuals will add to the burden of administering a waiting list, as they will have already been assessed and treated by a therapist within the department within the time limits set by the commissioners. Repeating such a process is frustrating for the patient and therapist alike, especially if the difficulty revolves around the treatment length having been too short for it to have been effective in promoting lasting psychological health, despite the treatment modality having been correctly selected and administered. If such individuals can be identified, for example through the application of the outcome measures routinely used in some departments (Clinical Outcomes in Routine Evaluation or CORE system of tools and patient satisfaction questionnaires – see http://www.coreims.co.uk and Barkham *et al*, 2001), or by outcome measures resulting from clinical governance work, including the present audit, then this gives scope for the delivery of psychological therapies to be tailored to these individuals, to promote lasting psychological recovery.

Standards

There are few national standards in this area and little published research to guide service provision. However, local guidance is widely available regarding areas such as waiting lists for treatment, where targets are commonly set and where 'payment by results' is highly relevant for commissioners and service providers in psychological services departments. Owing to the lack of available standards, this audit will allow benchmarking, in order to gather information about the existing service and to set standards, such as expected levels of re-referrals to the service, for future audit and to guide service development.

Method

Data collection

A list of patients who had been referred to the psychotherapy service was compiled from records regarding psychotherapy screening. These patients' records were for previous psychotherapy treatment of 20 sessions or fewer.

Data analysis

The number of patients re-presenting to psychological services after 20 sessions of psychodynamic psychotherapy was calculated as a percentage of total referrals to the service.

Resources required

People

This audit can be completed by one person.

Time

This audit will take approximately 4 hours.

Results

Of referrals accepted, 12.5% were re-referrals of patients who had received 20 sessions of treatment and a further 9.4% were re-referrals of patients who had received 21–30 sessions.

There had been some anxiety within the service that 20 sessions of psychotherapy would not be enough, particularly for patients with complex or deep-seated psychological difficulties. The results of this audit were therefore somewhat reassuring; however, it may be premature to draw firm conclusions, as this was the first round of the audit.

Recommendations

▶ A re-audit should be undertaken.
▶ Therapists working within the service should be surveyed to ask about their experience of delivering 20 sessions of psychodynamic psychotherapy, looking at details such as modality of psychodynamic psychotherapy used, client satisfaction, therapist satisfaction and action taken after completion of therapy.

Barkham, M., Margison, F., Leach, C., et al (2001) Service profiling and outcomes benchmarking using the CORE-OM: toward practice-based evidence in the psychological therapies. Journal of Consulting and Clinical Psychology, 69, 184–196.

Department of Health (2004) Organising and Delivering Psychological Therapies. The Stationary Office. Available at http://www.dh.gov.uk/en/Publicationsandstatistics/Publications/PublicationsPolicyAndGuidance/DH_4086100 (accessed October 2010).

100. Psychotropic prescriptions in dual diagnosis

Shankar Kuchibatla and Hany George El-Sayeh

Setting

This audit may be relevant in dual-diagnosis clinics or any in-patient ward with service users who have substance misuse problems.

Background

It has been noted that the prescription of psychotropics in patients with substance misuse problems infrequently meets the national gold standards. Psychotropics, when taken concomitantly with illicit substances or substitution treatments for substance misuse disorders, can cause physical complications (Lingford-Hughes *et al*, 2004).

Standards

The standards of the current audit were based on the guideline issued by the British Association of Psychopharmacology on depression and substance misuse (Lingford-Hughes *et al*, 2004).

▶ Patients with established depression and alcohol misuse and dependence should be prescribed selective serotonin reuptake inhibitors (SSRIs), and tricyclic antidepressants should be avoided in such cases.

▶ In the case of depression with opioid dependence, again, SSRIs are preferred, and tricyclic antidepressants should be avoided.

▶ The SSRI antidepressants are recommended as first-line pharmacotherapy for the treatment of comorbid anxiety with alcohol misuse and dependence.

▶ Atypical antipsychotics are favoured over typical antipsychotics for the treatment of schizophrenia with comorbid substance misuse disorders.

▶ Benzodiazepines are not recommended for the treatment of anxiety in patients who misuse alcohol or who have a history of alcohol misuse.

Method

Data collection

All medical records of psychiatric patients who had been reviewed in the drug and alcohol clinic were examined for entries and documentation relating to patient demographics, substances used, associated comorbidities, the psychotropic prescribed and the indication for its use.

Data analysis

The percentage of patients who met each of the above standards was calculated. The data were displayed as bar graphs and pie charts.

Resources required

People

It is suggested that this audit is undertaken by at least two people, owing to the large amount of information to be obtained for data analysis.

Time

The data collection itself may take up to four sessions. The data can be obtained over a few weeks. Primary care doctors may need to be contacted to gather information on the psychotropic usage by the patient.

Results

▶ Approximately 30% of the patients with substance misuse problems had comorbid psychiatric conditions.

▶ Of the comorbid illnesses, 78% were depression, anxiety or mixed anxiety and depressive disorders.

▶ In comorbid depression, the prescribing standard was adhered to for only 38.5% patients, as tricyclic antidepressants were used instead of SSRIs.

▶ The indication for the use of an antidepressant (anxiety or depression) was not clear in 32% of the cases.

▶ Only 20% of the benzodiazepines were prescribed for insomnia or anxiety. There was no clear documentation from primary care services on the indications for benzodiazepine prescriptions.

▶ Atypical antipsychotics were used appropriately to treat psychotic disorders in 67% of patients with comorbid psychosis.

Recommendations

▶ Awareness of the guidelines on prescribing psychotropics in comorbid illnesses with alcohol and substance misuse among community drug and alcohol teams should be increased by circulating the guidelines to staff.

▶ The communication between primary and secondary care staff needs to be improved, with a particular emphasis on updating the physicians concerned of any changes to the patient's prescriptions. Regular meetings between community drug and alcohol team staff and general practitioners could aid communication.

▶ The indication for psychotropic use should be clearly documented in the psychiatric case notes.

▶ A re-audit should be undertaken in 12 months.

Lingford-Hughes, A. R., Welch, S. J. & Nutt, D. J. (2004) Evidence based guidelines for the pharmacological management of substance misuse, addiction and comorbidity: recommendations from the British Association for Psychopharmacology. *Journal of Psychopharmacology*, 18, 293–335.

101. Rapid tranquillisation

Bethan Davies and Emma Court

Setting

This audit is relevant to all acute in-patient services where high proportions of patients are acutely disturbed and present a risk to themselves or others.

Background

The use of rapid tranquillisation for acutely disturbed patients is at times necessary to ensure the safety of themselves or others. Documentation of the reasons for its use and commensurate physical health monitoring are vital to ensure patient safety and to facilitate improved ongoing care.

Standards

Standards were obtained from the guideline on the management of violence from the National Institute for Health and Clinical Excellence (NICE) (2005) and the *Good Medical Practice* guidelines (General Medical Council, 2009). Of particular relevance were the following:

▶ The intervention selected must be a reasonable and proportionate response to the risk posed by the services user.
▶ At all times, a doctor should be available to quickly attend an alert by staff members when rapid tranquillisation is implemented.
▶ Medications should be prescribed and administered as per *Good Medical Practice*.
▶ The prescriber and medication administrator should pay attention to consent.
▶ The physical health of patients should be monitored as per the rapid tranquillisation algorithm.
▶ Any incident requiring rapid tranquillisation should be recorded using a local template.
▶ A post-incident review should take place as soon as possible and at least within 72 hours of an incident ending.

The target is that these standards are met for all patients who have received rapid tranquillisation.

Method

Data collection

All medication charts were reviewed for a 4-week period to determine who had been given any p.r.n. medication relevant to rapid tranquillisation (e.g. haloperidol, lorazepam or olanzapine). Oral medication was included only if it was given as part of rapid tranquillisation. A pro forma was used for data collection and the medical notes of these patients were examined to find the entries documenting the following:

▶ 'severe imminent' risk to self or others
▶ whether a doctor was contacted
▶ what medication was administered

233

- whether consent had been given
- any physical health monitoring carried out after rapid tranquillisation
- completion of local rapid tranquillisation monitoring form and incident form
- whether there had been a debriefing with the patient within 72 hours of the incident.

Data analysis

The results of the data collection were calculated in percentage terms and compared against a 100% target for each of the above standards.

Resources required

People

It is suggested that this audit is undertaken by at least two people, owing to the amount of information collected.

Time

For a service with 30 patients within an acute psychiatric hospital, it is estimated that the data collection would take 4 hours.

Results

- All the patients who required rapid tranquillisation had medication in intramuscular form.
- Documentation of medication administered and consent was excellent; however, the documentation of physical health monitoring and post-incident reviews was poor.
- Despite reference to local rapid tranquillisation forms and incident forms being completed, these were not located in the current medical notes.
- Filing of physical health monitoring forms was variable, and so data collection was incomplete.

Recommendations

- Documentation of all aspects of rapid tranquillisation (indication for its use, administration and follow-up) is required to ensure patient safety.
- Training for all staff involved in rapid tranquillisation needs to be carried out to ensure their familiarisation with the rapid tranquillisation algorithm, policy and local documentation requirements.
- A standardised location is required for the storage of all rapid tranquillisation documentation within the medical records so that information can be easily reviewed.

General Medical Council (2006) *Good Medical Practice*, paragraphs 1–3 and 20–22. GMC.

National Institute for Health and Clinical Excellence (2005) *Violence: The Short-Term Management of Disturbed/Violent Behaviour in In-patient Settings and Emergency Departments* (CG25). NICE. Available at http://guidance.nice.org.uk/CG25 (accessed October 2010).

Appendices

Appendix 1. Forms for section 136 of the Mental Health Act

Communication and monitoring information: form 1, completed by police (for police, patient notes & monitoring)

Station code	
Custody number (if applicable)	
Police reference number	

Please fill in the required sections and, where there is a text box (☐), put a Y (yes) or N (no) in the box.

Person detained – Surname:		Forename(s):	
Address:			

Place of birth:		Date of birth:	(DD/MM/YYYY)
Gender:	ID code:	Self-defined ethnicity code:	
PNC & local check done? Yes ☐ No ☐		PNC outcome:	
Date of detention: (DD/MM/YYYY)		Time of detention: (xx:xx hrs)	
Place of detention:			

Notes of incident/arrest

Since detention, has the person received any medical attention prior to arrival at a place of safety?
Yes ☐ No ☐ If 'Yes', please describe

Risk factors the place of safety or assessment staff should be aware of? (consider self-harm, suicide, physical aggression, impaired judgement, self-neglect, absconding, etc.)

Has the person been restrained? Yes ☐ No ☐ If 'Yes', how and for how long?

Is the person suffering from the effects of drink or illicit drugs? Yes ☐ No ☐ Unknown ☐

Initial Place of Safety used: S136 suite ☐ emergency department ☐ police station ☐

other (describe) ☐

If not S136 suite, explain: no S136 suite locally ☐ S136 suite full ☐ physically unwell ☐

too disturbed ☐ other (state) ☐

Ambulance requested at:	Date: (DD/MM/YYYY)	Time: (xx:xx hrs)

Conveyance to Place of Safety: ambulance ☐ police vehicle ☐ other (describe) ☐

If not ambulance vehicle, explain: person too disturbed ☐ patient too distressed ☐

would take too long ☐ other (describe) ☐

Arrival at Place of Safety:	Date: (DD/MM/YYYY)	Time: (xx:xx hrs)

Has the person been searched? Yes ☐ No ☐

Time of departure (police):	(xx:xx hrs)	Received by:	
Officer reporting (signature):		Wt. no.:	

Communication and monitoring information: form 2, for patient notes and monitoring

Person detained – Surname:				Forename(s):		
Rights leaflet was given and rights read at:	Date:		(DD/MM/YYYY)	Time:		(xx:xx hrs)

Professional	**Contacted at:**			**Arrived at:**		
	Date (DD/MM/YYYY)		**Time** (xx:xx hrs)	**Date (DD/MM/YYYY)**		**Time** (xx:xx hrs)
AMHP						
First Doctor						
Second Doctor						

If there were any delays, please state the reason on the next page.

Details of relative or friend

Name:	
Address:	
Tel. no.:	Informed? Yes ☐ No ☐

Assessment completed at:	Date:	(DD/MM/YYYY)	Time:	(xx:xx hrs)
Patient discharged from Place of Safety at:	Date:	(DD/MM/YYYY)	Time:	(xx:xx hrs)

Was the first doctor approved under Section 12 MHA?   Yes ☐   No ☐

Is the person on medication?   Yes ☐   No ☐   Unknown ☐

Any Serious Untoward Incident following detention including in place of safety? Yes ☐   No ☐

If Yes, please complete one of boxes and give details:

Minor self-harm ☐   self-harm requiring medical attention ☐   assault ☐   absconsion ☐

other (please state) ☐

Details:

Transfer from one Place of Safety to another Place of Safety prior to S136 assessment being completed   Yes ☐   No ☐

Name of unit:

Arrival at second place of safety:	Date:	(DD/MM/YYYY)	Time:	(xx:xx hrs)

Reason for transfer:

Was there a further transfer?   Yes ☐   No ☐   If yes, record above information on back of form.

Arrangements made after initial assessment

Was not suffering from mental disorder and was discharged ☐

Was suffering from mental disorder and was discharged but:

a) no follow up was required ☐

b) follow up was arranged ☐

Was admitted or transferred on an informal basis ☐

or under MHA section 2 ☐   3 ☐   other ☐ (please state)

To:	Ward:		Hospital:	
Arrival on ward:	Date:	(DD/MM/YYYY)	Time:	(xx:xx hrs)
Signed: (person completing form)			Print name:	
Date:		(DD/MM/YYYY)	Time:	(xx:xx hrs)

Appendix 2. Pharmacological management of alcohol withdrawal

Alcohol detoxification

Alcohol dependent patients exhibiting withdrawal features or at high risk of developing withdrawal (based upon their history) should be prescribed benzodiazepines. Dosage should be individually titrated against severity of withdrawal symptoms and signs. Individuals should normally remain in-patients until detoxification regime is complete.

Daily alcohol consumption	15–25 units		30–40 units		50–60 units
Starting dose of chlordiazepoxide	15–25 mg		30–40 mg*		50 mg*
Day 1 (starting dose)	15 q.d.s.	25 q.d.s.	30 q.d.s.	40 q.d.s.*	50 q.d.s.*
Day 2	10 q.d.s.	20 q.d.s.	25 q.d.s.	35 q.d.s.	45 q.d.s.
Day 3	10 t.d.s.	15 q.d.s.	20 q.d.s.	30 q.d.s.	40 q.d.s.
Day 4	5 t.d.s.	10 q.d.s.	15 q.d.s.	25 q.d.s.	35 q.d.s.
Day 5	5 b.d.	10 t.d.s.	10 q.d.s.	20 q.d.s.	30 q.d.s.
Day 6	5 *nocte*	5 t.d.s.	10 t.d.s.	15 q.d.s.	25 q.d.s.
Day 7		5 b.d.	5 t.d.s.	10 q.d.s.	20 q.d.s.
Day 8		5 *nocte*	5 b.d.	10 t.d.s.	15 q.d.s.
Day 9			5 *nocte*	5 t.d.s.	10 q.d.s.
Day 10				5 b.d.	10 t.d.s.
Day 11				5 *nocte*	5 t.d.s.
Day 12					5 b.d.
Day 13					5 *nocte*

*Doses of chlordiazepoxide in excess of 30 mg q.d.s. – should be prescribed only in cases where severe withdrawal symptoms are expected, and the patient's response to treatment should be regularly and closely monitored. Doses in excess of 40 mg q.d.s. should be prescribed only where there is clear evidence of very severe alcohol dependence. Such doses are rarely necessary in women and never in the elderly, or where there is liver impairment.

Liver impairment

The metabolism of benzodiazepines may be reduced in those who misuse alcohol because of liver impairment, which can lead to over-sedation.

Over-sedation

If the patient is very sleepy or over-sedated, the dose may need to be reduced.

Severe withdrawal or delirium tremens

Additional doses of oral chlordiazepoxide or intramuscular diazepam 10 mg may be necessary initially.

Severe behavioural disturbance

In-patients who do not respond to a benzodiazepine, haloperidol 5–10 mg orally or intramuscularly may be added.

Vitamin prophylaxis

Indication	Prophylaxis required
Incipient Wernicke's encephalopathy (confusion plus ataxia and ophthalmoplegia)	Two pairs of high-potency Pabrinex (vitamins B and C) ampoules t.d.s. for 3 days, followed by one pair daily for 3–5 days, depending on response
At-risk (significant weight loss, poor diet, signs of malnutrition)	One pair of high-potency Pabrinex (vitamins B and C) ampoules daily for 3–5 days
Lower risk	Oral thiamine 100 mg q.d.s., plus vitamin B compound, strong, 1 or 2 doses a day during detoxification

High-potency Pabrinex (vitamins B and C) can be given intravenously or intramuscularly. Anaphylaxis is a rare but recognised complication, hence facilities for treating anaphylaxis must be available. When giving high-potency Pabrinex intravenously, it should be diluted in 50–100 ml sodium chloride 0.9% or glucose 5% solution, and given over 10–30 minutes.

Printed in Great Britain
by Amazon